RWBB   ROGER WILLIAMS COLLEGE LIBRARY
RA790 .W518 1984
Wicks, Robert J
Counseling strategies and intervention t

3 1931 00065 5570

09-BTO-144

counseling strategies
and intervention
techniques for the
human services

DATE DUE

JUL 13 1996			
NOV 5 1996			

DEMCO 38-297

counseling strategies and intervention techniques for the human services

second edition

ROGER WILLIAMS COLLEGE LIBRARY

Robert J. Wicks and Richard D. Parsons

Graduate Program in Pastoral Counseling
Neumann College
Aston, Pennsylvania

LONGMAN

New York & London

RA
790
W518
1984

4-15-87

Counseling Strategies and Intervention Techniques for the Human Services

Longman Inc., 1560 Broadway, New York, N.Y. 10036
Associated companies, branches, and representatives
throughout the world.

Copyright © 1977, 1984 by Longman Inc.

All rights reserved. No part of this publication may be
reproduced, stored in a retrieval system, or transmitted
in any form or by any means, electronic, mechanical,
photocopying, recording, or otherwise, without the prior
permission of the publisher.

Developmental Editor: Nicole Benevento
Editorial and Design Supervisor: Thomas Bacher
Production/Manufacturing: Ferne Y. Kawahara
Composition: Graphicraft Typesetters
Printing and Binding: Malloy Lithographing Inc.

Library of Congress Cataloging in Publication Data
Wicks, Robert J.
  Counseling strategies and intervention techniques for
the human services.
  Bibliography: p.
  Includes index.
  1. Community mental health services.   2. Psychiatric
nursing.   3. Psychiatric social work.   I. Parsons,
Richard D.   II. Title.
RA790.W518   1984   362.2'0425   83–16240
ISBN 0–582–28471–6 (pbk.)

Manufactured in the United States of America
Printing: 9 8 7 6 5 4 3 2 1   Year: 92 91 90 89 88 87 86 85 84

The importance of the role played by the "significant others" in the development and maintenance of the emotional well-being of each person has been emphasized in this book. We have been very lucky to have many of these important people in our lives who have consistently provided us with the caring, sharing, and helping needed for our own growth. By dedicating this book to our brothers: RONALD and RAYMOND—JOSEPH and JACK, and our sisters: NOEL and MEG— ANN and BEVERLY, we acknowledge their special significance in our lives.

contents

appendixes
159

a
counseling keystones
161

b
glossary of psychological and psychiatric terminology
182

preface

In 1977, when the first edition of this text was written, the preface opened with the statement: "Community psychology has finally come of age...." Not only was the statement an accurate reflection of the state of community psychology in the late 1970s, but it was clearly prophetic of the essential role community psychology has come to play in all of our lives in the 1980s.

A number of significant social changes have occurred that have impacted the delivery of mental health services. The late 1970s saw a greater emphasis given over to the early detection and treatment of emotional problems. Further, the number of allied health professionals who were providing mental health services increased, as did their levels of sophistication and interest in ongoing professional development.

The increased sophistication of these professionals paralleled the development of college and institutional training programs for allied health professionals, as well as the prominence of courses dealing with practical psychological concepts occurring within human service curricula. Even with this increased opportunity for training, the need for trained professionals increased at a faster rate than the supply of well-trained mental health professionals. This demand for mental health services has stimulated interest among a number of professionals, associate professionals, and community workers such as physicians' assistants, nurses, caseworkers, teaching staff members, and other human service personnel, to develop the skills necessary for properly and efficiently intervening. The second edition of this text has been designed to help meet the needs of these individuals.

Counseling Strategies and Intervention Techniques for the Human Services is designed to provide material on behavioral theory and application in a practical format. By offering information from varied, and sometimes not readily available sources, the text attempts to introduce readers to a number of critical issues, with the hope that they will be encouraged to read further. The goal of this book is to increase the reader's awareness of the information-gathering process, the basic elements of the helping relationship, and the methods employed by allied health professionals in treating emotional disorders.

The second edition attempts to increase both the breadth and depth of the material covered by the previous text. Increased breadth is provided by material on preventive mental health services and on the process of consultation. Further, each of the chapters was revised, not only to reflect the current literature, but also to deepen discussion of the various topics by including a behavioral/cognitive theoretical focus in addition to the more traditional psychodynamic one.

Following a brief introduction to the historical and philosophical evolution of the current state of mental health services, the reader is introduced in part one to the diagnostic–problem identification process. Chapters 1 to 3 have been devoted to the presentation and discussion of typical information collection procedures employed by the Human Service Worker. Specific attention is given to the interview process, the Historical and Mental Status Evaluation and the general issue of Psychological Testing.

Part two of the text presents a general rationale for the need and value of classification systems (chapter 4) and describes the specific utilization of such a system for the analyses of anxiety (chapter 5) and depression (chapter 6). These two specific syndrome patterns were selected for in-depth presentation since they are not only two of the most frequently encountered problems, but have demonstrated that they can lead to the development and exacerbation of almost all other emotional and medical problems.

Part three provides an overview to the strategies and procedures employed in the intervention and treatment of emotional and behavioral problems. Attention is given to identifying the essential ingredients of all such helping relationships. Further, each of the chapters within this part elaborate upon the need to provide interventions that foster prevention as well as remediation.

The final section (part four) outlines the importance of knowing how to communicate with other individuals who play significant roles in the process of treating and preventing emotional problems. Special attention is given to the process of report writing (chapter 10) and interacting with other professionals in a consulting relationship (chapters 11, 12). It is hoped that these chapters will strengthen the reader's understanding of some of the less obvious problems and limitations to treatment, and encourage them to value the importance of community collaboration and involvement.

In essence this second edition, like its predecessor, is directed to those nursing, mental health, educational, and community health personnel, as well as other human service workers, who often serve as the first line of problem identification and intervention, and who thus need and want to know more about the causes and treatment of emotional problems.

As was the case with our previous works, this volume could not have been completed successfully without the support and technical advice of our wives—Michaele Wicks and Karen Parsons. Further, we wish to recognize all of those professionals who have so greatly influenced our own professional development and whose influence is evidenced throughout this text. Finally, we would like to thank Ann C. Wood, our typist, whose pleasant style and willingness to be flexible has enabled us to meet our project deadline.

Robert J. Wicks
Richard D. Parsons

introduction

The field of human services and mental health delivery is entering a new era. Now, more than before, an ever increasing demand for services will fall on all too few service providers. Consumer sophistication and demand for accountability is on the increase. The requirement for services aimed at fostering personal growth instead of merely focusing on remediation is a new standard being set. To suggest that we are entering an era of mental health revolution appears quite valid. This revolution seems to be one that is progressing from an emphasis on mental health delivery toward an emphasis on primary prevention. Like its predecessors, this revolution will shake the very philosophical foundation upon which much of the field of human service is founded. The specific thrust of such a revolution or shift in paradigm can best be understood in light of the history from which it has emerged.

This introduction will attempt to provide an overview of the origin of this revolution and detail the specific implications that such a revolution holds.

Revolutions in Human Services

Primary prevention, which represents a radical change in the approach to the delivery of mental health services, can still be conceptualized as a logical extension of the other major historical developments in the field of mental health. Consequently, to fully appreciate the timeliness of the current revolution, the "science" of mental health—with its sometimes sordid past—needs to be understood.

Humanizing the Mentally Ill. The *first revolution* occurred in Paris in 1792. The conditions surrounding the institutionalization of the insane at that time were miserable and inhumane. "Treatment" as we now know it didn't exist. This first of the mental health revolutions resulted in literally removing the chains from the insane. It gave birth to the notion of mental

1

illness as a human condition, rather than as a manifestation of demonical possession. The person behind the movement was Philippe Pinel (1745–1826). His radical inclusion of kindness and fresh air in the treatment regimen of the mentally ill was a complete change from the previously dark period when such persons were "hanged, imprisoned, tortured, and otherwise persecuted as agents of Satan" (Deutsch, 1946). Primitive practices such as trephining (i.e., drilling holes in the head to allow the demons to escape), dunking, exorcism, and burnings were prescribed as attempts to rescue the afflicted person from the grips of the demon rather than providing remedial or preventive approaches to the problem of mental illness.

Thus, a dramatic shift into the Age of Enlightenment occurred when Philippe Pinel "freed" the chained and enslaved inmates of La Bicetre in 1792. This unchaining marked, not only an upgrading of treatment procedures, but also a major shift in the perception of the insane. Instead of being characterized as less than human (demonical), they were seen and treated as *people* whose illnesses were neither supernatural nor untreatable. Further, this philosophical shift provided a new level of respect for those who might be interested in researching the causes of, and treatment for, such conditions. It was this "coming out" and acceptance within the scientific community that fostered the growth of the second revolution.

Introducing the Clinical Model. The *second revolution* occurred with the advent of Sigmund Freud's work on the unconscious. Freud (1856–1939) demonstrated that some people suffering from mental illness could be cured through a verbal interchange. In addition, Freud's extensive work on the nature and working of the psyche provided the impetus for viewing mental illness as an entity falling well within the realm of the natural and one that could be "scientifically" investigated, understood, and treated. Freud's early observations moved the field of mental health into an era of the clinical model, a model that posited as one of its major tenets that an inappropriate or abnormal behavior was symptomatic of an underlying "disease." The cause of this disease was posited as being reflected in the intrapsychic (unobservable, interior) conflict that arises out of an imbalance among the forces in the personality; Freud named these the "ego," "id," and "superego." (See appendix B.) However, although Freud had a positive influence on the strategies and techniques used by the human service professional, his focus on treating mental illness from a medical or clinical paradigm was to also forestall attention to the role played by interpersonal and social factors in both the incidence and form of mental illness. Furthermore, the long-term, one-to-one treatment that was conducted by professionals extensively trained in psychoanalytic technique, prevented easy multiplication and extension of services. Few were qualified to be "analysts" and, in turn, very few were fortunate enough to receive help.

Not only was the efficacy of Freud's therapeutic model criticized, but the validity of Freud's "disease" orientation itself soon came under fire. The cause and effect aspect of the medical model was questioned by psycho-therapists in the 1950s and early 1960s, using conceptual models based on learning theory (Krasner and Ullman, 1965; Wolpe, 1958). It was from such questioning and criticism of the direct-service (one-to-one), clinical (under-lying disease) model that the third of the revolutions in human services sprang.

The Community Model.   The *third revolution* was marked by the develop-ment, in the 1960s, of *comprehensive* community mental health centers in the United States. The hope was that any person needing help with emotional problems (no matter what level of severity) could be served through one treatment center. This extended the notion that had been developing throughout the first two movements. It highlighted the basic humanity of those with emotional problems and the apparent continuity between the "sane" and the "insane." The focus that emerged from this third revolution was that *all* people in need can and should benefit from mental health services and thus deserve to have access to them (Parsons and Meyers, in press). The new orientation emphasized: (1) a community rather than clinical orientation; (2) prevention rather than therapy; (3) a readiness to experiment with innovative, short-term remedial strategies; (4) uses of new sources of manpower (e.g., paraprofessionals, educators, parents); (5) a commitment to client and community control of mental health policy rather than professional control; (6) identification of environmental stresses present in the community that could cause mental health problems; and (7) indirect service rather than direct service delivery (Bloom, 1973).

At the very heart of this community movement was the desire to provide services to the greatest number—which included not only those in distress, but also those who might be prone to problems such as depression, anxiety, stress, etc. Thus, in addition to providing direct, one-to-one service, those involved in this third revolution began to turn to more indirect methods of service delivery (e.g., consultation, community educa-tional service, etc.) as a means of providing the greatest good for the greatest number. It was this shift in emphasis to an indirect mode of service delivery that was one of the most significant impacts of this revolution in human services. The focus on indirect service delivery had a number of implications for the helping profession. For instance, if new manpower sources (e.g., paraprofessionals) were to be used, they would require support via short-term, in-service training, and follow-up consultation. Further, the enlightened community control of mental health policy demanded ongoing communication between professionals and community groups. This third revolution began to shift the focus of human service professionals from being solely concerned with remediation to addressing the ways and means of prevention.

This shift in focus away from an aim of providing service to those in need (i.e., remedial), to one in which the goals were the fostering of growth and a decrease in the danger of the development of mental health problems (i.e., prevention), marked the fourth and current revolution in human services.

A Focus on Prevention. As understanding of the causative factors involved in mental illness and adjustment problems increased, the search for increasingly sensitive tools for early detection soon followed. Concerns about ecology, environment, and extrapersonal factors affecting one's mental health and psychological adjustment began to take the forefront and remain of essential concern during this *fourth revolution.*

This shift in orientation from a concern about mental health deficiency (i.e., searching for a person's psychopathology) to a concern for mental health growth and facilitation signals the need for a redefinition of the role and function of the human service professional. Such a redefinition marks an expansion of responsibilities to cover *all* people who currently experience mental health or adjustment difficulties, along with all those who in some way carry a high risk of experiencing such difficulties in the near future. It demands that human service professionals expand their service delivery in order to include strategies for prevention, along with those current practices aimed at remediation.

Levels of Prevention

A number of authors have distinguished between the various levels of prevention (primary, secondary, and tertiary); and although the view of this introduction is that primary prevention is the most desirable, each level of preventive service has a role to play in our delivery of human services and will thus be presented for consideration.

Primary prevention can be defined as an approach including efforts designed to prevent the occurrence of a disorder in a particular population by promoting the emotional well-being of all of those in that particular group or community. Although it is generally agreed that primary prevention is designed essentially to prevent the development of mental health disorders, the actual specifics of how this is to be accomplished is open to much discussion and debate. However, what appears consistent throughout the literature and in the discussion surrounding the issue of primary prevention is that such prevention can be accomplished through a number of ways that share certain common characteristics. Primary prevention techniques, for instance, include the following goals: (1) to decrease the incidence of new cases of emotional disorder occurring in the population rather than to prevent a particular individual from becoming mentally ill; (2) to inhibit the harmful effects of stress and other factors in the environment that can create mental health problems; (3) to promote environmental conditions that support positive mental health; and (4) to build competence and coping skills that foster mental health (Parsons and Meyers, in press).

Although it is clear that the already overtaxing demands placed upon the mental health/human services professional leave little time and energy for consideration of primary prevention strategies, prevention as a focus can still be a reality for the human service professional. Granted that primary prevention often demands political, economical, and social resources that may fall outside the boundaries of the human service profession, secondary and tertiary levels of prevention are clearly within the resources available to the human service professional and thus need to be considered as essential to the intervention strategies employed by this profession.

Secondary prevention becomes necessary when primary prevention strategies don't totally succeed. It focuses on problems that have already begun to appear. The goal of secondary prevention is to shorten the duration, impact, and negative effects of the disorder. That is, the goal of secondary prevention is to intervene in such a way as to prevent the occurrence of the "typical" cycle of the illness and thus prevent it from reaching a point of severity. Therefore, it employs early identification and early treatment regimens as a means of achieving its preventative goals. If this approach is not used or is unsuccessful, the third level of services, *tertiary prevention*, is used. This method includes those techniques designed to reduce the consequences of severe dysfunction after it has occurred.

Tertiary levels of prevention appear to be the form of prevention most often applied by today's human service professional. In contrast to a direct remedial focus, tertiary prevention attempts, not to only remediate the presenting problem, but also to provide the means of developing a more adaptive (preventive) coping style in the future. Yet, while providing a needed remedial and preventative value, tertiary prevention is still primarily a reactive orientation in which the human service professional waits for the presentation of the disorder before reacting with strategies for intervention.

New Demands—New Skills

Not until the fourth revolution do we as human service professionals move away from the reactive position and begin to take leadership in helping to remove the extrapersonal factors affecting mental health problems and increasing the coping/adaptive styles of all. The call to lead requires that we begin to reduce our use of direct-remedial and tertiary prevention services, and begin to increase our utilization of secondary and primary prevention strategies. Thus, although human services have been legislated to meet the demands of those in need, human service professionals need not wait to intervene until these problems have reached full manifestation. Rather, as a necessary outgrowth of human service delivery, they can begin to employ early detection screening of potentially high risk populations and intervene to reduce the potentially negative impact of the disorders prior to their reaching severity. Preschool and early childhood developmental screening, pre- and paranatal parent training, hotlines and crises intervention services, are all strategies that need to be employed by the human service professional as a means of promoting early, effective intervention.

The fourth revolution is truly challenging human service professionals to reflect upon their role definitions and professional orientation in order to reach far beyond their typical foci to include the goals of primary prevention in their intervention strategies. Along these lines, a number of theorists have begun developing three apparently productive strategies for promoting such primary prevention.

Focus on Social Environments. For example, the current interest in the analysis and modification of social environments (e.g., Moos, 1973; 1974; 1975) appears to be one area in which strategies are being developed to enable mental health/human service professionals to achieve primary prevention in their service delivery. Work on the analysis of social environments has begun to indicate specific factors (e.g., degree of autonomy, degree of affection) manifested in a variety of social environments (e.g., school, work) that contribute to increasing mental health problems. Moreover, this work has led to the development of instruments for early detection and modification of potentially harmful social environments.

Focus on Competence. A second line of research that has special import for the human service professional in his or her search for techniques and strategies that promote primary prevention, is that of addressing the issues of developing competence and adaptive capacities. A variety of extensive training programs aimed at increasing the participants' interpersonal cognitive problem-solving skills, social adaptive ability, assertive skills, and stress management abilities are now being developed. Such training programs reflect the essential nature of primary prevention. They demonstrate that in addition to remediating problems, the human service professional needs to provide service to those who are not in need of remediation, but who seek personal growth. The theory of this *preventive* orientation is that increased personal growth and competence will in turn help to prevent the development of mental health problems (Spivack and Shure, 1974; Allen et al., 1976).

Focus on Stress Reduction. With the increasing research demonstrating the effect of environmental stress in the creation and maintenance of emotional problems, stress reduction techniques have emerged as a third set of strategies to be used by the human service professional attempting to achieve primary preventing goals. Stress reduction techniques seek to reduce the impact of environmental stress (e.g., loss of job, change in marital status, bereavement) by increasing the person's capacity to recognize early signs of stress and more effectively cope with or manage such stress. For example, social support systems such as parent support groups, drug and alcohol hotlines, runaway hospices, etc., serve to reduce the potential negative effects of these stressors and assist people in coping more effectively with the stress they encounter. These social support systems also emphasize the development of early detection procedures to help individuals. Anticipatory guidance, stress innoculation, and anxiety reduction are examples of techniques that have been used by human service professionals in attempting to accomplish the stress reduction goals (Phillips, Martin, and Meyers, 1972).

The current inclusion of a preventive focus to the role of the human service professional now requires that such professionals be trained not only in direct service techniques (i.e., diagnostic and counseling strategies), but also in certain procedures (e.g., consultation strategies) that facilitate the modification of those social-environmental conditions and procedures that foster the development of mental health problems. Chapter 11 will discuss the process and format for mental health consultation. However, its relationship to preventive goals is briefly described here.

Consultation

Consultation involves six essential ingredients: (1) it is a helping or problem-solving process; (2) it occurs between a professional help-giver (the consultant) and a help-seeker (consultee) who is responsible for the welfare of another person (the client); (3) it is a voluntary relationship; (4) it attempts to share in solving a work problem; (5) its goal is the resolution of the current work problem; and (6) the impact of the help-seeker works in such a way that future problems may be handled more sensitively and skill-fully (Meyers, Parsons, and Martin, 1979).

The purpose of including consultation as a form of service delivery for the human services is not to argue against direct service delivery or even to suggest that one form of service delivery is better than another. Rather, the intent here is to demonstrate that as human service professionals we need to be prepared to offer a broad spectrum of services ranging from one-on-one direct contact (e.g., counseling, testing, psychotherapy) to the more indirect forms of service delivery, as might be found in organizational consultation.

If a bias is being expressed it is that consultation is a method that will facilitate human service professionals in their attempt to include preventive foci among the services they render.

Consultation, by definition, attempts to provide an educative element in the service delivered. This is done so that a generalization or "transfer effect" might be noted. This effect is not only the most important goal of mental health consultation (Meyers, 1981), but one that also signals its value as a preventive service. Through the principle of generalization the consultee is encouraged to apply the processes and procedures developed for remediating a particular work problem to the solution of future problems. Therefore, regardless of the immediate effect on the client or consultee, the educative environmental focus of consultation dictates that there will be a long-term effect that will impact not only the referred client (remedial), but also all other potential clients experiencing that environment (preventive). In other words, if the consultee's behavior or environment changes significantly, it is possible that the changes will have a positive impact on clients who have not yet demonstrated problems and thus will help prevent the development of such problems in the future.

Levels of Consultation

The consultation model described in this book (chapter 11) posits four different levels of intervention. Levels I and II provide more or less direct service to the client. Level III consultation provides service to the consultee (who in turn will affect the client). The goal of this form of consultation is to change the behavior, attitudes, and/or feelings of the consultee, with the hope that such modification will result in changes for the client as well. Level IV consultation (service to the system) provides the most indirect of all service to the client. The goal at this level of consultation is to improve the organizational functioning of the system as a whole. Thus the impact on the specifically referred client will be filtered down through the various system interventions inaugurated. It will not only impact this particular client but also all those within the system.

At the levels of service to consultee (level III) and service to the system (level IV), the goals of primary prevention appear to be best achieved. Service to the consultee can facilitate the consultee's influence on the mental health of all of the clients for whom the consultee is responsible and thus may serve as a primary prevention strategy. For example, consider a situation in which a teacher (a consultee) requests assistance from a human service consultant regarding a problem child (client). When the consultant can help the consultee (the teacher) recognize that the particular client's (student) negative behavior was due to the consultee's classroom management style and further assist the consultee (teacher) to modify his/her classroom management techniques, not only will the presenting problem be ameliorated, but potential future problems of a similar nature and genesis can also be avoided. Under such a condition the consultant not only provided a remedial service, but by providing the consultee with a mechanism for assessing and modifying his/her professional style assisted the consultee in becoming more effective in facilitating the mental health of all present and future students (clients).

The level of consultation or service to the system (level IV) also has obvious implications for primary prevention. Systems-oriented consultation, through its focus on organizational structure and/or processes, produces changes in the system that in turn will affect the mental health of the consultees and clients in the system. Thus a system that is highly authoritative, is overly demanding, and employs threats or coercive methods of control will most certainly impact the mental health and adjustment of those attempting to work within the system. Further, the consultant who intervenes in such a way as to move the organization toward a more participatory form of governance and the creation of a work atmosphere characterized by professional respect and positive regard will have taken giant strides in not only remediating the emotional problems of those experiencing difficulty within the former system, but also in providing system changes that may help prevent similar problems from emerging in the future.

Summary

The field of human services is truly moving into a new era, an era that springs naturally from its own historical roots. From the moment Phillipe Pinel unchained the inmates at La Bicetre, the mental health field was placed on a trajectory that would lead it to a position wherein services are aimed not only at remediating, but also at preventing mental illness.

The inclusion of a preventive focus in the realm of the human services demands that human service professionals develop a set of consultative skills in addition to their more typical direct service skills. They should no longer be satisfied with "simply" remediating a problem with which they are presented. Rather such professionals must begin to take an active stance—attacking the sources of mental health problems—and in so doing provide the primary prevention service demanded of the fourth revolution.

This was a brief introduction to the historical foundation of the fourth revolution in mental health services. With this introduction as a base, the remaining chapters will comprise an overview of the specific skills and functions demanded of the human services professional.

part one

diagnostics

problem identification

1 / *interviewing*

Regardless of the focus of the human service professional or the demands of the presenting problem, at the heart of all human service interventions lies the existence of a *helping relationship*. The quality of this relationship is the "key" to the success or failure of the intervention strategies applied.

All too often human service practitioners, in their eagerness to assist their clients, rush into the performance of their duties (testing, counseling, or referring) without giving proper consideration to the type and quality of relationship that they have established. Nowhere is such lack of concern for the quality of the interaction evidenced as it is in the oftentime rigid, mechanistic interview style of the neophyte mental health worker.

To even the most talented, motivated, and serious worker, conducting an interview can be a challenging endeavor. Productive interviews result from interactions between clients and interviewers who have the ability to exploit their personal talents through the application of soundly based interpersonal techniques.

To become an adept interviewer, one must (1) acquire an appreciation for the complexity of the process of human communication; (2) develop the skills and attitude necessary for a facilitative reception and expression of the information; and (3) become familiar with the specific characteristics of the therapeutic interview. Though a knowledge of the qualities and techniques of interviewing is not more important than being an empathetic, understanding person, an awareness of the interview process will enable an individual to develop personal interviewing skills more easily. Thus, the worker will find a study of the interview process an essential aid in obtaining the information needed to help a client through a crisis or in assisting the client to reach a decision.

What Is an Interview?

An interview is a basic process of communication in which two or more persons interact to achieve some goal. Essentially, it is a purposeful conversation.

Unlike an ordinary conversation, an interview is goal oriented. But it should not be approached as an interaction in which the interviewer appears with a pencil and paper and makes a "shopping list" of the client's problems or complaints. Instead, an interview is an interpersonal encounter in which the interviewer aims to put the interviewee at ease in order to gain a clear understanding of his or her reason for appearing at the clinic, hospital, or office.

The goals of the interview vary in different settings. In a psychiatric unit the object may be to explore a patient's mental status, the environmental factors (home, occupational) affecting his life, and the characteristic ways in which he deals with the world.

In a lawyer's office the objective may be to weigh a client's chances of winning a lawsuit through an examination of the elements in her favor. In a hospital it may be to determine the symptoms the patient is manifesting and the previous treatment received. Or a personal interview may aim to determine the suitability of an applicant for a particular job. In this instance, the interviewer would measure the job description against the applicant's experience and abilities to estimate his or her probable future performance.

As we have noted, interviewing goals vary depending upon the type of setting and the professional framework in which the worker operates. However, whatever the objective—whether to determine the cause and extent of an emotional or physical disorder, or a session with other aims—every interview is purposeful.

Further, each interview, regardless of its setting and purpose, is influenced by the unique nature of the elements composing it; that is—the interviewer, the interviewee, and the *process* of communication between them.

The Interviewer

The interviewer is first and foremost a message receiver. It is the principal intent of each interviewer to gather and accurately process information about the client that is received through this goal-directed communication process.

The therapeutic communication process—both at the level of information reception and problem assessment (the interview), and remediation and intervention (counseling)—is a complicated, sensitive process that demands one's complete and *active* attention. Many of us, however, have been trained even from childhood to be passive, polite, quiet listeners. Interviewing, while most certainly a polite process, is far from being a passive one. The good interviewer must not sit back and simply absorb the information provided by the interviewee. Rather, the interviewer needs to reach out and actively listen and involve himself or herself in the data-gathering process of an interview. As noted, such active involvement requires that the interviewer *attend* to the interviewee.

Attending—Physically and Psychologically. Attending or "being with" another requires both a physical position and a psychological orientation. Gerard Egan (1977), for example, pointed out the importance of one's body orientation to the accurate reception of information during a face-to-face encounter such as an interview. Following Egan's observation, it is suggested that, when in the process of an interview, the interviewer take and maintain an attentive body orientation. This orientation can be characterized as being face to face, straight, open, slightly forward in a leaning position, with the maintenance of eye contact, and relaxed. Such a SOLER (straight, open, lean, eye contact, relaxed) position will not only ensure the receptivity of the interviewer, but help convey to the interviewee that one is "really with" him or her in this moment. One need only experiment with talking to a person who fails to maintain eye contact, or stands askew, to appreciate the value of the SOLER posture.

In addition to taking an actively receptive physical stance in the interview, the interviewer must be psychologically active in the communication exchange. All too often we sit back and attempt to absorb the information supplied by the interviewee. However, such passive listening often leads to moments of inattentiveness, moments in which the listener escapes into daydream or simply fades out because of the boredom of the moment or the massiveness of the information supplied.

In order to avoid this nonattendance, the interviewer needs to become an active-empathic listener. That is, the interviewer needs to reach out and attempt to step into the world of the interviewee, so as to experience that world as he/she experiences it. Such active listening is a *total* listening: a listening to all of the signals (verbal and nonverbal, explicit and implied) being sent by the interviewee. Further, such active listening requires that one check reception for accuracy by providing the client feedback regarding the message as it was received. It requires that the interviewer separate the messages sent by the interviewee from those that are self-generated. An accuracy check might be obtained by simply asking the interviewee, "Is this what you mean?" or stating that "it seems that you are feeling (saying, implying, etc.)". This can prove to be a powerful tool to ensure interviewer receptive accuracy.

To further ensure that the client's statements are interpreted in the most objective manner possible, interviewers must constantly question their own motives and reactions when processing data during and after sessions. For example, when conducting an intake interview in a mental health setting, if a young male should be questioning a client of his own age and with a similar background, he would need to take care not to avoid or cut short the discussion of topics about which he is sensitive. If, for instance, the interviewer had smoked marijuana, he might be tempted to avoid the topic with the reasoning, "Marijuana isn't so bad; after all, even I smoke it once in a while." However, by avoiding mention of this subject, he may fail to discover that the patient smokes thirty "joints" of marijuana daily, resulting in social, occupational, and possibly legal difficulties.

In reflecting on their own styles of interaction with the client, interviewers must also be constantly alert to their personal responses to a client's critique of them. When blame or anger is directed by the client toward the interviewer, the interviewer must analyze both the criticism and personal feelings about the criticism. When praise is offered by the client, similar self-questioning is advisable. In both instances, reactions to the personal evaluations made by the interviewee may cause an emotional reaction that will obscure the cause of the criticism or praise.

Though the client's comments may be reasonable, the interviewer should try to discover whether they are made for the purpose of changing the subject or diverting the interviewer's attention from the client's anxiety.

The following interaction (during an extensive medical intake interview between a student physician's assistant and an alcoholic) illustrates how a patient may try to verbally abuse the health professional to change a train of thought and questioning.

> *Physician's Assistant:* "How often do you drink alcoholic beverages?"
> *Patient:* "You're pretty nosey. What kind of question is that to ask? Are you saying I'm some kind of drunk or something?"
> *P.A.:* "To ensure that we get a complete picture of your physical health pattern, we are concerned with the kind of food you eat and beverages you drink."
> *Pt.:* "You're just a young student. Why don't you practice your stuff on some other guinea pig?"

In this case, if the P.A. should become angry and defensive, little progress would be made. When, by means of anger or praise, the client changes the topic being discussed, the interviewer should mentally note sensitive areas that may prove to be closely related to the client's problems. In the case of the P.A. and the alcoholic, the P.A. has sensed the seriousness of the problem. If an individual becomes angry or evasive when questioned about drinking habits, it is likely that alcohol has, for that person, become "a friend worth protecting and hiding." (Once an alcoholic reaches a certain stage, he or she will attempt to conceal the extent of the addiction, no matter how obvious it may be that alcohol abuse is a serious problem.)

Interviewer Preparation.   Interviewers may avoid being caught off guard and reacting poorly to surprising or personally unpleasant information revealed by the interviewee if the client's personal situation is understood beforehand. Seeing the world as the client does is an essential aid to mutual understanding.

If a health professional is interviewing a male adolescent with his first case of venereal disease, there are some things that should be expected. For example, if the interviewer in this instance expects the youth to be somewhat fearful, causing him to react with hostility or in an anxious fashion, there is less chance that the interviewer will respond thoughtlessly to an angry outburst by the youth during the intake interview. Also, understanding the sensitive nature of the situation, the interviewer will take special care to see that the session is held in strict privacy.

The Interviewee

Response Styles. The type of responses given to an interviewer's questions provide clues to the client's way of dealing with his/her world. When under stress, there are five major ways an individual may react. These are fairly straightforward in most cases and will reveal themselves if the worker is alert to their potential impact. These categories of adjustment to stress are regression, avoidance, suspiciousness, depression and bravado.

Regression is encouraged in many inpatient settings. The client is tended to, often uninformed as to the treatment being administered, is usually requested not to be very active, and is frequently clothed in hospital garb and identified by a bracelet placed on the wrist. However, in some mental health therapeutic communities, this is changing. The patient is instead encouraged to be as responsible and involved as possible, and is informed as treatment proceeds.

The dependent type of client is quite at home in a situation that encourages regression, readily accepting the submissive patient role. Dependent clients see the interviewer as one who can be relied on for help and eventual cure.

Those who use *avoidance* as their key defense against being made uncomfortable by the stress of an emotional or physical illness try to put any questions or anxiety-laden issues out of their minds. Evasiveness and oversimplified responses are the tactics used by the client to arrive at a simple solution to his or her problem. Health personnel are expected to carry full responsibility for a cure without complications or excessive discomfort.

Suspiciousness is a common reaction among general hospital and community mental health patients. Such clients consider illness as confirmation that they will have problems when they rely on others for advice as to how they should live their lives or what medical precautions should be taken to avoid illness. These clients also project their own feelings of aggression onto others; in expecting others to be hostile to them, they attempt to get a step ahead of their "aggressive acquaintances" by being cold or hostile to them first.

As might be expected, such hostile behavior keeps others at a distance, confirming the client's conviction that other people are at fault. Awareness of this style of dealing with the world will help the interviewer to prevent the client from being abandoned interpersonally.

Depression is the natural response of any emotionally or physically incapacitated person. However, some individuals may become lethargic and react to stress in a helpless or hopeless fashion as a matter of course; depression and hopelessness are their chief means of dealing with the difficulties that arise from being ill or disturbed (see chapter 6, "Depression").

Bravado is another common reaction style to the stress of a health problem. Instead of feeling insecure and threatened by an illness, which naturally generates some dependency, the person puts such feelings out of consciousness (repression) and exhibits the opposite to what is in fact felt (reaction formation). Rather than becoming dependent and closely following medical prescriptions or accepting the idea that some self-examination may be in order, the client takes all responsibility, occasionally to the point of disregarding or flaunting professional advice.

Bravado that conceals fear can be extremely dangerous. In one instance, a patient who suffered a heart attack (myocardial infarction) dealt with his fear of dying by manifesting counterphobic behavior that could have resulted in his death. Counterphobic behavior may be defined as actions taken by individuals to show others that they are masters of their fear. In the case of the man with a fear of dying from a heart attack, counterphobic behavior took the form of his going into the bathroom and doing pushups until he provoked the symptoms of another attack.

People deal with physical and emotional illnesses in many ways. The interviewer who notes the particular style in which a client is reacting already has a good deal of information as to how this person will handle the side effects or difficult outcomes of his or her incapacitation. Certainly, awareness of such patterns is useful if the health professional is to gain an understanding of the client in a short time, which is most often the limitation an interviewer must operate within. (And this is usually the situation in community mental health and hospital settings, where prolonged contact is often impractical or impossible.)

Silence and Nonverbal Communication. Earlier in the chapter the importance of body language (SOLER) in conveying the message of "being in attention" to the client was noted. The importance of this body posture was stated to be that it not only set the mental stage for the interviewer to become fully attentive, but that it also conveyed this attentiveness to the client, thus facilitating his/her disclosure. Nonverbal messages can often provide clues to the underlying feelings one is experiencing at the moment and thus can prove invaluable sources of data to the perceptive interviewer. For example, just as the interviewer attempts to signal openness and receptivity to the others' messages by being face to face, straight, and open (e.g., legs uncrossed), so too does the client who assumes that body posture. However, if the interviewer begins to note a shifting in the client's posture, a turning away, or closing up (e.g., crossing his/her arms tightly across the chest or intertwining his/her legs, somewhat uncomfortably, yet protectively), then the interviewer may be correct in assuming that the client is feeling defensive at this point in the exchange.

One of the ways that interviewers can determine a client's style of reaction is by observing nonverbal signs, particularly during periods of silence in the interview. Clients may become silent at normal breaks in the communication as they wait to see what the interviewer wants to know next.

However, individuals may become silent during an interview for other reasons. The interviewee may be embarrassed, angry, or confused, or be attempting to see how the interviewer is going to react to something said, resulting in a silent response. If interviewers are alert to nonverbal communication, particularly during silent periods, they will be able to note clients' messages and react appropriately, or take stock for future use when normal communication resumes.

In today's noisy world, it is difficult for many to remain silent when others stop speaking. We are accustomed to constant sounds, and a good conversationalist who can talk on various topics when others fall silent is held in high regard.

However, effective interviewers must become accustomed to silence. They must learn to be active listeners when the interviewee is talking, as well as when he/she suddenly falls silent. It is the poor listener who waits anxiously for the chance to talk; the interviewer must therefore never show this kind of anxiety.

In active listening, interviewers are carefully noting what the interviewees are saying verbally and nonverbally, as well as simultaneously monitoring their own nonverbal reactions to this information.

Monitoring one's own nonverbal communication is very important. Often an interviewer may react in a negative or surprised manner, thus revealing personal feelings about the information received. When this happens, the interviewer must be alert to such nonverbal slips, or he or she will fail to understand why the client subsequently tries to hide similar information for fear of rejection or retaliation.

The Process

The Encounter—Initial Anxieties. First impressions are not only the most lasting but the most influential in terms of governing a process of interaction. Quite often the interviewee entering the initial interview is unclear as to what he/she might expect. Under such a condition of "not knowing," the client often generates a number of anxiety-provoking expectations about the course and outcome of the interview. Similarly, the interviewer, being unclear as to what to expect from this client and this interview, may experience anticipatory anxiety prior to engaging in the actual interview.

Such negative expectations and anxious concerns about the interview process often develop from an individual's concerns about his/her own ability to perform. The client and the interviewer may find themselves concerned about issues such as: "Will the other like me?" "Will I be able to respond completely?" "What happens if I fail or make a mistake?" Further, clients often have unrealistic expectations about the power and ability of the mental health professional: "Will he be able to read my mind?" "Will I have to lie on the couch?" "Can he commit me?" etc. Such unrealistic expectations and concerns, if allowed to continue throughout the interview, can prove quite detrimental to the entire interview process. As such, steps need to be taken to properly structure the initial contact so as to remove these negative expectations.

From the point of the initial contact or greeting, the interviewer needs to convey the message that I (the interviewer) am a friendly, caring, supportive professional and that this (the interview) will be a safe, confidential, productive encounter. Simple actions such as smiling, going out to meet the client (as opposed to waiting for the client to come to you), and structuring the interview environment so that it is a relaxed, comfortable setting may all go a long way to convey the desired positive tone of the interview and therefore ameliorate many of the client's initial negative expectations.

In addition to such social amenities, the interviewer can allay a number of the client's concerns and assist in creating a positive interview atmosphere by a number of preplanned interview techniques. For example, during the initial stages of the interview, the interviewer should provide a brief overview to the goals and process to be followed. Stating that "...we will spend the next thirty minutes sharing some information about the (job/problem/course of treatment/etc.) and try to come to some common agreement as to what goal we hope to achieve" will help provide the client with guidelines about what to expect in the interview. Such guidelines will help reduce the anxiety often experienced by a client entering this unfamiliar encounter.

Besides providing an overview, the interviewer should describe the "rules" of the interview; that is, what will each participant be expected to do and what topics will be covered. The interviewer needs to make clear that the interview is an *exchange*, not an interrogation; that it is *confidential*; and that the client if *free* to respond in whichever way he/she so desires (i.e., there is no absolutely right/wrong answer).

Such structuring during the early stages of the interview not only conveys to the client that the interviewer is competent and professional, but will also serve to reduce the initial fears with which the client entered the relationship.

Questioning the Interviewee. When the art of questioning an interviewee is mastered, the amount of information obtained can be impressive. Moreover, the client's anxiety level can be kept quite low while the data-gathering operation proceeds. Questions can be posed in ways that express interest ("Could you tell me more?") or the need for clarification ("How did you think that happened?") or even direction ("Could we pursue that a bit more?"). All of the aforementioned uses of questioning are truly valuable in the hands of an experienced interviewer. However, questions demanding justification ("Why?") or those creating a climate of interrogation need to be avoided.

The client enters the session with an agenda, a desire to express some issue or concern. Perhaps the primary responsibility of the human service professional, at this point, is to be sure not to prevent or block the client. As such, an interviewer needs to be skilled in asking "open" questions.

Open questions are those that invite the client to expand, elaborate, or expound on a point rather than simply ask for yes or no answers. It is often in an expansion of the original presentation that real insightful data are obtained.

Open questions allow the client the opportunity to provide direction to the interview. "Closed" questions (i.e., those that can be answered with a simple yes or no, or a few words) often create a condition in which the client feels as if he/she is being "machine gunned with rapid fire interrogation." Further, closed questions require the interviewer to completely structure the interview. Such structuring often creates an interview with a question/answer format and limits the information acquired to that specifically requested. This is not to imply that the use of closed questions is entirely unwarranted. Their use is often essential when the interview is aimed at obtaining clearly defined, factual information. What we are suggesting, however, is that a tightly structured interview often falls short when the concern is the unveiling of the client's feelings, unique personality, or distinctive orientation. It is under these conditions that open questions prove most beneficial. Open questions have also been found to be suitable for beginning an interview ("What would you like to consider today?"); stimulating the client to expand on a point ("Could you tell me more about this?"); or even helping the client focus on his/her feelings about an issue ("How does talking about this make you feel?"). By providing the interviewee the freedom to respond as he/she wishes, the interviewer avoids the possible danger of inappropriately using questions to place the interviewee in a defensive posture.

While we are suggesting that open questions are valuable in that they provide the client with the needed freedom of self-expression, we are not implying that an interview should be an aimless interchange of idle chatting.

Possibly the most basic rule from which all other rules concerning questioning are derived is that questions should be purposeful. The following diagram illustrates the goals of questioning in a medical setting when the interviewer is trying to establish a client's pathology:

Single question: symptom
Group of questions: syndrome

If medical interviewers are to determine the disease a person is experiencing, questions should be designed to elucidate individual symptoms. Separate symptoms can then be grouped into a pattern that reflects the client's pathological syndrome.

Though such a medically oriented interviewing diagram illustrates a restricted goal, it emphasizes the principal rule of effective questioning: *All questions should relate to a plan or goal.* Questions should be designed to expand or explore particular topics when important information is missing, when the client is confused or evasive, or when the interview strays from its objective.

In general, questions should be clear, simple, brief, purposeful, logical, on a level the interviewee can comprehend, and presented in a conversational manner. More often than not, counselors are dealing with people under emotional and/or physical stress. If questions do not follow in a logical progression, are phrased in a stilted manner or in psychiatric jargon, or contain too many elements, the interviewee may become confused and will certainly have difficulty answering satisfactorily.

As with most rules, there is a major exception. In some instances, when dealing with an extremely sensitive area, the interviewer will wish to conceal his or her train of thought. This will avoid arousing harmful anxiety in the client by disguising the reason or object behind a particular line of questioning.

For example, if the interviewer wishes to know about a client's intake of drugs, this area might be discussed in the context of questioning the client as to what medicines are normally taken. In this way, the client is not alerted to the interviewer's concern with the relationship that drug taking has to his or her health problem. Instead it will appear that the interviewer accepts the fact that many people normally and naturally take certain drugs when under stress, or in certain social situations when they feel "a bit tense."

Even though the interviewer may ask the question in a neutral, nonconfronting manner, the client's answers may be inadequate or marked with emotion. When this occurs, the client should not be scolded or criticized;

rather, the interviewer should reflect upon the possible cause of the unsatisfactory reply.

In some cases a person may answer with hostility because a question is in fact quite blunt or because it has been misinterpreted. A client may not reply fully to a question because of confusion about its meaning. The reasons why an answer can be less than expected are numerous and varied.

One easy test to see if the form of the question is the cause of confusion or hostility is to come back to the same area later in the interview with a question differently phrased and, if possible, more indirect and neutral than before. However, whether it turns out to be the topic itself or the way the question is phrased, the important point to remember is not to show annoyance when a person does not answer satisfactorily. Much can be learned by further reflecting and employing appropriate techniques when an inadequate or emotional response is evoked by a question.

Transitions. The interviewer's adept use of a smile and warm greeting, attending posture, and open questions will ensure that the client is willing to disclose information freely. As a result of setting the stage for a facilitative interview, the interviewer may find that a wide variety of topics are touched upon. The interviewer may then come to a point in the interview at which he/she desires to explore another topic or a particular topic in more detail.

If the interviewer moves about without an awareness of where the session is going or with little consideration for the client who may become confused or threatened by a surprising move into a new subject area, anxiety can be greatly increased. For this reason, interviewers should be aware of the use of different types of transitions.

During the session the interviewer can make the transition from one topic to another in three ways: smoothly, clearly, or abruptly. The *smooth transition* occurs when the client is permitted complete freedom in the choice of subjects to be discussed and the length of time for discussion. Though this permits clients wide liberty and encourages communication, it is usually impractical in medical or mental health settings to allow clients proceed without some guidance.

Since health workers are usually pressed for time and most explore a number of medical or psychiatric areas to avoid missing an important factor that could adversely affect the client's health if left unnoticed, the *clear transition* is most frequently employed in hospital and community health facilities. This type of transition involves three steps:

1. Interruption
2. Clarification
3. Topic change

The following excerpt from an interview conducted by a mental health worker trainee with a new patient illustrates the process. In this interaction, the worker has decided she has enough information on the patient's drug history and wants to discuss his previous employment.

> *Mental Health Worker:* (Interruption) "Excuse me a minute Mr. Graham, but let me see if I understand what you've said thus far." (Clarification) "You say that you have used. . . ." (Mental health worker briefly reiterates the information she has received to see if the patient wishes to change or add to the impression given; once this is done, both are ready for the next phase.) (Topic change) "I wonder if we could spend some time now on some of the jobs you've had in the past several years?"

In using the clear transition, the interviewer creates an opportunity to move the session along while at the same time evaluating the impressions received from the client. The use of *clarification* (step 2), not only encourages the client to correct information incorrectly received by the interviewer, but provides the client with evidence that the interviewer is truly "with" him/her in this session. Further, providing clients with such clarification can help them pull together their thinking and feelings about the issues discussed. This closure not only gives clients a sense of satisfaction about coming to some form of task completion, but prepares them for the movement to the next topic.

In preparing for transition, the interviewer needs to remember that the intent of the clarification is to provide the interviewee with the *essence* of what has been said and not the exact words or phrases. All too often the novice interviewer, intent on "getting it right," concentrates so hard on mentally rehearsing the interviewee's words, in preparation for the point of clarification, that he/she misses the subtle look, inflection, or tone that demonstrates the essence of the client's message.

The primary danger in using clear transition centers on *timing.* If the interviewer interrupts too soon or too often, pertinent data may be lost. Thus, the decision to stop the flow of communication on a topic should be made when it is obvious that the client is being redundant or is needlessly expanding on a particular area.

An *abrupt transition* is rarely used. However, it may be appropriate and effective in avoiding or preventing an increase in a client's anxiety level. If during the session a client becomes upset over a particular topic and the interviewer feels that the client's anxiety level is too high to explore an area further, the topic can be abruptly changed with a plan to return to it later in the session or at another time. On the other hand, when dealing with an antisocial, difficult youth who displays a complaisant, uncooperative attitude, abruptly switching from topic to topic may help to elicit information vital to the preservation of life itself, as in the case of a drug addict with other serious medical problems.

Confrontational Messages.   When attempting to discuss appropriate confrontational styles in human service interviews, *the interviewer/helper must overcome the general tendency to equate the word "confrontation" with that of a destructive, aggressive, hostile act.* Within the context of a helping relationship, confrontation represents an invitation by one participant in the interview to the other participant, to look at, discuss, clarify, or reconsider some events occurring within the interview.

For example, we have all had occasion while talking with a friend to question a point they made in relation to which we had contradicting information. For example, imagine the following dialogue between two mental health workers.

> *Mental Health Worker:* "Gads, how are we ever going to get through this paper work, especially now that they are cutting back on our student assistant?"
> *Co-worker:* "I'm not sure, but I think the memo said the students would finish at the end of this term, so I guess we still have some help for at least two more months."

The above example provides an illustration of a simple *didactic* (informational) confrontation—a confrontation in which one member of the dialogue (co-worker) invited the other (mental health worker) to reconsider his/her position in light of this more accurate information (didactics). Needless to say the same type of confrontation (i.e., didactics) could have occurred with quite different results if the co-worker had responded ("Just like you, dope! You never read anything. The memo we got said the students stay the semester.")

Confrontation, therefore, happens anytime we call to question another's behavior, attitude, or feelings. Since confrontation is inevitable, one needs to attempt to provide for productive, facilitative, and relationship-building confrontations. For a confrontation to be productive and constructive in the helping relationship, a number of factors need to exist. First, the relationship should be viewed by the participants as a helping, caring, supportive relationship. Secondly, the motivations of the confronter should be those of seeking clarity and growth in the relationship rather than attempting to demonstrate power or one-upmanship. Finally, the style of confrontation should be characterized as descriptive and tentative rather than judgmental and accusative (Parsons and Meyers, in press).

The interviewer who can descriptively and tentatively point out areas of client misinformation (as with the example of the mental health worker and the memo) or mixed and confusing messages (e.g., "He says he's interested, but he is always late.") can constructively move the interview to a greater level of accuracy and clarity.

Privacy and Professionalism.   The interviewer must be sensitive to the possibility that the interviewee is not used to, or comfortable with, personal disclosure and consequently might feel quite vulnerable in the interview. An interviewer must therefore be alert to remain professional and respect the client's privacy at all times.

Even if an interview is very informal and, of necessity, is held in a corridor or a community mental health dayroom, the interviewer should try to move to that part of the area that offers the most privacy. This point cannot be overemphasized. Too often, particularly in health settings where professionals conduct many assessments, interviewers may become insensitive to the importance of privacy when conducting an interview.

The interviewer may feel that since the information being obtained is *only* about such *innocuous* topics as "educational background," "marital status," "age," etc., confidentiality need not be emphasized. This same interviewer, however, needs to consider his/her own experiences when being asked to respond about areas that he/she finds personally sensitive (e.g., drinking habits, salary, political affiliation, etc.) to appreciate that the sensitivity of an issue rests not in the topic covered, but in the eye of the disclosurer.

Summary

Once the interview has nearly completed its course, the interviewer should end the session with a real sense of closure and without leaving the client up in the air. If the situation is one in which only one interview is scheduled, the client should be permitted final questions and given prescriptive or referral information that may be appropriate prior to terminating the session. On the other hand, if the interview is one of a series, in many instances the client's last minute questions may be deferred to a later session.

Once the interview is ended, careful notes about it, together with comments on the significance of important points, are useful. In this way, data are recorded and decisions about immediate steps (i.e., referral) can be made without delay.

Such observational or anecdotal notes should be extensive. Feelings, points of behavior, or words expressed that at first appear to have little relevance or importance to the central issue might later prove to be the essential link to the understanding of the client's responses.

For example, the session might have become difficult at some point because the interviewer stumbled into a sensitive topic. Or the interview might have been poor throughout because of the attitude of the interviewee or the interviewer.

After considering the reasons for the session's unproductiveness, an additional point should be considered. The interviewer must devise measures or strategies to avoid another unsatisfying session at a future time.

(In some cases, the unproductivity results from the interviewer setting goals that are too high, too soon; and it may be overlooked that each new interviewee is a stranger with his or her own personality differences and attitudes.)

Finally, the interviewer needs to examine his or her personal opinion of the client if the session does not appear to be productive. This is essential because if the interviewer, at some level of consciousness, blames the client for the lack of interpersonal progress, future encounters will be adversely affected.

Interviewing is a difficult task. Yet, whatever the level of difficulty, the interview is an important process, and health professionals should give close attention to the development of interviewing skills. Effective and successful interaction with the client is critical to the attainment of the goals of health professionals.

2 / *historical and mental status interviews*

Administrators in hospitals, clinics, schools, and community settings often seek the help of health professionals on the mental health team to conduct psychiatric assessments of new clients requesting or referred for care. The initial evaluation phase in an institutional or community setting may be quite extensive, involving a series of physical examinations, psychoneurological tests, and interviews. On the other hand, it may consist of only a brief contact screening interview; such an interview usually aims to quickly assess the immediate needs and complaints of a hospital patient or a client requesting treatment in a community mental health center.

General Approach

One of the most frequent criticisms of interview procedure guidelines for conducting historical and mental status interviews has been that they emphasize the importance of identifying the *areas* of investigation, while deemphasizing the value of being aware of the *process* of investigation. In other words, the message conveyed by most manuals on conducting assessment interviews has been "the information must be gotten at all costs!" One might assume that narrowly focused and rigid questioning was the proper means to secure accurate data.

While it is true that much of the literature on psychiatric interviewing was not intended to convey such a message, unfortunately many mental health professionals have so interpreted manuals and books. This problem often arises when a psychology intern, mental health worker trainee, or new psychiatric resident conducts the intake interview at a diagnostic conference. In a diligent effort to obtain a great *quantity* of material, the novice interviewer may proceed to cross-examine the client in the manner of an attorney in the erroneous belief that this is what is expected and is in the client's best interests.

Perhaps this problem is an inevitable part of the process of learning to be a humanistic and sensitive interviewer, as well as an efficient one. However, by our examination of the problem here, some occasions for potential injury to the client's feelings may be foreseen and avoided.

With this in mind, the remainder of this chapter will be devoted to guidelines concerning the information the interviewer should attempt to gather in conducting historical and mental status interviews.

However, what follows should not be taken as a rigid sequence of directions in conducting an interview. Instead, the interviewer should know the areas well enough to permit flexibility in moving from topic to topic in line with the client's train of thought. If one clearly knows the areas to be dealt with, the order of topics can be altered or patterned for each client without overlooking any major area that might provide important clues concerning the client's problem and his or her capacity to deal with it.

Changing Interview Models

As noted in the introduction, the past two decades have seen a revolution in mental health. One of the outcomes of this change has been to deemphasize the importance of the medical model of treatment. In turn, this has had a direct effect on the information-gathering processes used. In common with the medical model, which is concerned with the history or course of a disease (whether physical or functional) and the symptoms manifested, historical and mental status interviews were considered to be the best approaches to data gathering when dealing with a new client. The increasing tendency to avoid the medical model has naturally resulted in less emphasis on this traditional type of interview.

Some community centers have eliminated historical and mental status interviewing procedures entirely. Others retain them for use only when long-term treatment is being considered or when the consultant psychiatrist chooses to use them. However, many mental health settings—especially those working in conjunction with a medical center in which traditional methods persist—have changed their policy concerning who should conduct the interview.

Historical and mental status interviews formerly were conducted by a psychiatrist or psychologist. How recent changes in the mental health movement have changed this can be seen in the following quotation from the *Comprehensive Textbook of Psychiatry*:

Until quite recently, it was the physician who, by virtue of his training, was considered best suited to collect clinical data; but it became clear that it was far less important to insist that the clinician should always be a physician than it was to minimize those factors that can have an adverse effect on the interaction between the patient or other informants and the clinician charged with the task of obtaining the necessary information. The use of community workers has shown, for instance, that some patients can be put at ease if they know that the health professional gathering the data is a representative of or, at least, is familiar with the subculture in which the patient lives. (1975, p. 724)

Thus, although in some mental health settings historical and mental status interviews are being eliminated or employed only in specific situations, others, particularly those with medical affiliations, continue their use.

Where such methods are used, the health professional is most often charged with the responsibility of assisting in conducting interviews. Obviously, this new responsibility requires the associate professional in the health care setting to be now more than ever aware of the principles involved in conducting historical and mental status interviews.

Historical Interview

Ideally, a historical interview should reveal what place the presenting complaint has in the overall pattern of the client's life. In seeking information on aspects of the individual's past and current life style, the object is to determine in what ways the problem has influenced his or her daily life and, in turn, how environmental and developmental elements may have affected the cause and form of the reported difficulties. In this way, clues to etiology, duration, severity, and effectiveness in handling the problem can be discerned.

The Present Complaint. After basic data about the interviewee are secured, a detailed account *in the client's own words* is obtained. In this part of the interview, a wide range of information may be uncovered. However, a minimum requirement is to obtain answers to the following questions:

1. Why did you come to the hospital at this time?
2. How did you get here?
3. When did your problem begin?
4. How has the presence of your difficulties affected other aspects of your daily existence?

In reply to the first question the client should supply the reason for admission and the precipitating factor that made his or her problem worse.

This is the ideal time to see how much insight the person has concerning the complaint. Also, *specifics* in the description of the problem need to be elicited. For example, if the client should complain of being "up tight," further explanation should be sought. Accordingly, the interviewer may prompt the client to continue with a description of the complaint: "By 'up tight,' what do you mean?" "How did your 'up tight' feelings manifest themselves?"

Since the intent is to begin to develop the clearest, most specific picture of the presenting problem, it is helpful to have the client describe how the problem affects his *emotions/feelings*; his *ability to function and perform typical day-to-day behaviors*; and his *thoughts and thinking processes*.

How an individual was brought to the hospital is important for a number of reasons. If the client's family accompanied him or her, some estimate may be made of the degree of support that can be expected from the family. Do they intend to abandon the client or can they be counted on to take part in the rehabilitation process? Was the individual brought forcibly to the hospital or picked up on the street by the police? Is the client a self-referral, or did a physician advise him or her to come in? Among other things, these questions will reveal information that will help the interviewer to assess the client's self-reliance and motivation.

Knowing the circumstances concerning the most recent onset of the problem or complaint should provide some clue to the underlying reason for it. This may be less true in some cases than in others, but there are many types of disorders that develop or become more severe in response to an event that can be traced to an underlying dynamic etiology. For example, a self-referral at least indicates that the client has some perception that a personal problem exists. On the other hand, if a person is forced to seek help, he or she usually has a poor understanding that a problem exists, much less has motivation to correct it.

The interviewer needs to know a great deal about how the client's difficulties have affected his or her daily activities. Determining how the development of symptoms may have caused changes in occupational, educational, interpersonal, sexual, leisure, and health styles will show how and to what extent the individual has had to alter his or her way of performing daily tasks.

Information about the impact of symptoms may also expose any secondary gains the manifestations of the problem may produce. For instance, if an anxious executive becomes ill when given heavy responsibilities, he or she would not have to face the source of the anxiety since the illness would preclude coming to work.

Psychological and Medical History. The importance of knowing about a client's previous history of psychological problems and how they were treated is obvious. All periods of inpatient, outpatient, or private treatment should be recorded. The type of treatment used (group, individual psycho-therapy, psychotropic drugs, shock treatment, and so on) is important because it will help to determine the severity and diagnosis of the problem and indicate the kind of treatment, if any, that should be ruled out in the future.

It is generally advisable to acquire the names and addresses of the person(s) involved with the previous treatment. In addition, the interviewer should have the client sign a "release of information" form. This client permission will allow the interviewer to gather relevant information about the client's previous treatments, and thus measure the records against the client's memory and presentation of the experience. In addition it is often helpful to ascertain from family sources information regarding these previous episodes and treatments.

A complete medical and personal history covers more than the record of past illnesses and accidents. In addition to physical problems that resulted in surgical or outpatient treatment, the client should be questioned closely concerning personal habits and any chronic symptoms. These might include sleeping problems, enuresis, stammering, or convulsions, to name but a few (see table 2.1). It must be emphasized that overall assessment is concerned not only with major difficulties in the past, but includes all behaviors that might help in the formulation of a thorough initial understanding of the client and his/her assets and problems.

Family History and Current Environment. Family history should trace the client's family environment from birth to the present. Any changes (housing, moving from one place to another, deaths, and so on) or unusual stress is noted, in addition to basic chronological data concerning siblings and other family members.

The facts of family history will aid in determining the time and circum-stances of the initial onset of the problem, while more current information may help the interviewer to determine whether the client's present home environment is affecting his or her problem.

In addition to family circumstances, the climate at work or school may be significant. Psychological difficulties often stem from the stresses of work or education. On the other hand, resources may be found in the occupational or school setting that can be incorporated in the overall plan for treatment to improve the client's functioning as a worker or student.

Mental Status Interview

In a separate interview the client may be questioned with the aim of assessing general mental status. A mental status examination is an organized method for acquiring data essential for the BASIC understanding

Table 2.1. Historical Interview Outline

1. *Date and Place of Examination*
2. *Identification of Client*
   a. Name   e. Marital status and number of children
   b. Birth date (age)   f. Occupation
   c. Sex   g. Address and telephone number
   d. Race
3. *Current Complaint (Detailed Account)*
   a. In client's own words
   b. From other sources (family, friends, records...)
4. *History of Present Complaint*
   a. Why was help sought?
   b. When did problem begin?
   c. What was happening in the person's life during problem's onset?
   d. How has current problem affected person's life (interpersonal activities, sexual adjustment, occupation, leisure activities, characteristic ways of responding, family life, memory, sleep and eating habits, general activity level, concentration, personal dress and hygiene...)?
   e. Symptom development: description of current and previous functional and organic symptoms (location, times of onset, duration, and intensity).
   f. Secondary gain from symptoms: how patient has benefited from presence of symptoms (i.e., ulcer and sickness prevent executive from being promoted to position that would require more responsibility and work to do).
5. *Previous Mental Problems*
   a. Previous types of therapeutic treatment
   b. Effects of treatment
   c. Places of treatment
   d. Periods of incapacitation
   e. Neurological and psychophysiological disorders
6. *Medical History*
   (Normally not done by nonmedical personnel; this section usually completed by physician, nurse, physician's assistant, or associate professional with strong allied health background.)
7. *Personal History (Infancy to Adulthood)*
   a. Preschool milestones, reaction patterns, diseases, accidents, sicknesses, and emotional problems. These should include circumstances surrounding mother's pregnancy; eating, sleeping, and bowel habits and problems; childhood illnesses; medical complications surrounding teething, growth...; early emotional and behavioral problems, such as enuresis, stuttering, temper tantrums, hyper/hypoactivity, tics, convulsions, losses of consciousness...; methods of dealing with stress, such as withdrawal, aggression; and peer relations.
   b. School age (6 to 18) adjustment. This area includes peer adjustment; school history; alcohol and drug use during this period; sexual behavior and attitudes toward it; emotions and physical problems peculiar to this time; social adjustments outside of school; interpersonal style and problems with family.
   c. Adult adjustment. This area includes college and post high school education and training of any sort; occupational and vocational history; military;

activities, ambitions, and conflicts surrounding interpersonal relations on job; social and sexual adjustment; marital history, including courtship or period during which client was living with someone else prior to or in lieu of marriage; financial status and problems.

8. *Family History*

a. Description of various household members whom the client had contact with from infancy on; special attention is given to mother, father, and siblings.

b. The following historical and descriptive data should be included: birth/death dates of any household member; central conflicts, problems; positive elements; mental/physical illnesses; traditions; intellectual/personality/ethnic issues encountered in the family history.

c. Current data, including present status of family members and their dependents, independence or general relationship to client and other family members.

(Currently some interviewers spend a good deal of time exploring this area of family history because of the recent interest of many psychiatrists and psychologists in the role of the family in maintaining a patient in a sickness position.)

9. *Present Environment*

a. Detailed description of physical and psychological environment to which the patient will be returning.

b. Changes in job, finances, or home situation that might take place and need attention during outpatient treatment or hospitalization. (For example, who is supporting family? Who will ensure property is not stolen in rented room during long-term hospitalization?)

c. What problems will be present upon disposition or resolution to release client from care? (For example, will it be necessary to get client a room to live in instead of having him return home?)

10. *Physical Identification*

a. Interviewer's nontechnical impression of person being interviewed. (Is person fat, tall, gruff, sloppy, and so on?)

---

of the client's current situation, resources, and style of coping. BASIC is used here as an acronym for the types of information sought during a mental status examination.* The interviewer will closely note the individual's *B*ehavior and physical appearance, *A*ffect and emotional state, *S*ensorium or information reflecting the functioning of the client's central nervous system, *I*ntellectual functioning, and *C*ognitive Processes (see table 2.2).

Behavior and General Appearance. Information collected under this category provides the interviewer a clear "picture" of the client's conduct and style or manner of presentation. Information recorded includes the

---

* The organization of this section reflects the authors' adoption of the concept of BASIC ID presented by Arnold Lazarus (1981).

Table 2.2. Mental Status Examination/BASIC

1. *Behavior and General Appearance*
   a. Dress (overly neat, sloppy, bizarre...)
   b. Posture
   c. Gait
   d. Motor activity level (e.g., retarded)
   e. Attitude (cooperative, hostile...)
   f. Behavioral mannerism (tics, pacing...)
   g. Speech (monotonous, pressured, unusual aspects of it, aphasia, stuttering, slurring, relevance, pitch, level...)
2. *Affect and Emotional State*
   a. As reported by client
   b. As client appears to interviewer
   c. Duration, intensity, appropriateness, anxieties, swings...
   d. How emotionalism is handled
3. *Sensorium*
   a. Attention and alertness (understanding, responsiveness...)
   b. Orientation
      (1) Time
      (2) Place
      (3) Identity
   c. Memory
      (1) Recent
      (2) Remote
4. *Intelligence, Insight, and General Information*
   a. General fund of information
   b. Insight
      (1) Awareness of illness
      (2) Ability to report etiological, supporting, and personal factors involved in the development and continuance of illness
5. *Cognitions and Cognitive Processes*
   a. Speed
   b. Associative abilities (neologisms, word salad...)
   c. Organization
   d. Content
      (1) Disturbances: perceptual (hallucinations, illusions...), and thought (referential ideas, delusions...)
      (2) Productivity
      (3) Concerns (physical, environmental, obsessions, compulsions, anti-social, sexual...)
   e. Abstract thinking
   f. Judgment
      (1) Social convention
      (2) Planning, problem-solving abilities
6. *Summary of Findings*
7. *Diagnostic and Prognostic Impressions*
8. *Management and Treatment Recommendations*

client's demographic characteristics, such as name, age, address, marital status, and description of physical characteristics (e.g., height, weight, posture, obvious physical disabilities). Also recorded are descriptions of the client's gait, unusual or peculiar movements, tics, and expressive mannerisms, both verbal and nonverbal (tongue protrusion, lip smacking, blinking, etc.)

Affect and Emotional State. It is important to observe the client's emotional state or *affect* as the interview proceeds. The client's own assessment—whether, for example, he or she feels depressed or elated—should be compared with the interviewer's impression of the client's emotional state. Abrupt changes or inappropriate responses should be carefully noted. In addition to the evaluation of affect based on observation of nonverbal signs and the client's own report of his or her emotional state, questions may be asked to determine depth of depression, elation or another strong emotion, and the circumstances surrounding their occurrence.

Here are some sample questions:

Do you feel depressed (or have you felt depressed in the recent past)?
Do you ever feel life isn't worth living?
When was the last time you felt really elated?
What kind of things make you panicky and fearful?
Do _____ feelings last long?
What is going on when you start to feel _____?

Sensorium and Functioning of the Central Nervous System. Often questions regarding neurological impairment or organic brain dysfunction arise as part of the presenting problem. Throughout the mental status examination the interviewer should be alert to record evidence of impaired general alertness or consciousness, orientation, memory, and concentration.

Specifically, the interviewer should be attentive to any inconsistency or fluctuation in the client's ability to be responsive and alert throughout the interview. The interviewer needs to assess whether the client is oriented to person (his/her own name); time (hour, day, month, and year); and place (where he/she is, who he/she is being interviewed by...). Accordingly, and if not previously noted, the client is questioned directly as follows:

What is your name?
Where are you?
What day is it? What month? What year?

Recent and remote memory also are tested. Evaluation of remote and recent memory usually is based on the client's own historical data. However, immediate recall may be assessed through the use of a digit span or other memory technique.

For example, the patient may be asked to repeat a series of digits—4, 7, 10—after the interviewer. Then the same process is repeated, but the client is instructed to repeat the series in reverse. This task is presented very simply: "I am going to give you some more numbers. When I am finished, I want you to repeat them, but this time in reverse. For example, if I say 3–2–4, you would say 4–2–3."

Another method is to ask the client to memorize the names of four objects that he or she will be asked to recall later in the interview. Then, about halfway through the session, the client is asked to repeat the names of the objects.

Finally, the degree to which the client is able to concentrate needs to be assessed. If the client has responded accurately and fluidly to the interviewer's questions, then perhaps sufficient evidence of normal attention has been gathered. On those occasions on which the interviewer is unsure of the client's ability to concentrate, he or she can ask the client to perform basic arithmetical tasks, such as a "serial of sevens." The client can be asked to subtract by 7s from 100, as a measure of the client's ability to concentrate on simple, repetitive tasks.

Intellectual Function, Insight, and Fund of General Information. A quick estimate of a client's intelligence may be obtained by means of a series of general questions: "What are the capitals of Russia, England, and France?" "How far is it from New York to Chicago?" "How many nickels are there in $1.75?" "In what direction would you be traveling if you went from Chicago to Brazil?"

The mental status interview will also reveal insight into the causes, symptoms, and ramifications of being emotionally troubled. Some clients may deny having any problem at all. Others may have only a superficial or detached notion of their difficulties. Occasionally, however, clients will demonstrate a surprisingly accurate emotional and intellectual grasp of their situation. This area of discussion normally comes about naturally as the client is queried as to his or her reasons for being at the clinic or hospital.

Cognitions and Cognitive Processes. The form, speed, and content of expressed thoughts are usually accurate indicators of the state of cognitive abilities and judgment. Can the individual organize answers to direct questions? What is the rate of speech and problem-solving abilities? Are expressions and comments logical, conventionally acceptable, appropriate to the client's age, and generally understandable? Or do thoughts appear to be delusional and unproductive? Does the person hallucinate, are thoughts unproductive, possibly obsessional or antisocial?

Abstract thinking may also be impaired when mental illness is organically based. To determine whether an individual is able to conceptualize and generalize, and to avoid more concrete forms of reasoning, the client may be asked to interpret several proverbs or sayings:

What is meant by "People in glass houses shouldn't throw stones"?
What does "Don't cry over spilled milk" mean?
How would you interpret "One swallow doesn't make a summer"?

Summary

Once information is gathered from historical and mental status interviews, the interviewer after checking other reports—such as social work reports; laboratory, neurological, and psychological tests; or notes by nurses or attendants that may be available—measures those reports against the information supplied by the client.

After checking all of the data from institutional and home contacts, a full report is made concerning the items listed in tables 2.1 and 2.2. This information is followed by a summary of the findings and a diagnosis, prognosis, and list of recommendations for treatment.

As indicated earlier in this chapter, these kinds of interviews are no longer common in all settings. Even some medical settings—particularly those in community clinics—have eliminated the traditional historical interview.

However, variations of the interviews we have described remain common practice in most settings. In addition, there is a strong trend toward delegating the task of conducting such interviews to health workers who perform under the supervision of a medical or psychological director.

With these trends in view, this chapter has been designed to provide the health professional with the fundamentals of historical and mental status interviewing. Since clients and treatment settings vary, the material presented here is intended only as a tentative guide. Subsequent supervised experience and further reading will provide further amplification. The contents of this chapter offer the interviewer a guide that should enable him or her to move flexibly through the interview, while pointing out the important areas to be covered before the interview is concluded.

3 / *psychological testing*

At first glance, psychological testing would seem to be beyond the range of the human service worker's concerns. Just as drug therapy is a function reserved to the psychiatrist, intelligence and personality testing appears to be an activity limited to the clinical psychologist.

To some extent this is certainly true. After all, human service workers do not usually administer or interpret psychological tests. However, apart from these restrictions, there remains two reasons that make it important for the human service specialist to have knowledge of psychological testing.

First, human service professionals need knowledge about the "how," "what," and "why" of testing because they are implicitly involved in the testing process. Quite often it is the human service worker whose checklists, interviews, or observations serve as the first line of data collection. It is from this initial "testing" that diagnosis and decision-making processes begin to take form. As such, these preliminary measures and procedures (interviews, checklists, observations, etc.) need to be guided by the same "rules" applicable to the more standardized testing procedures.

Secondly, human service workers need to ask whether or not the questions they ask, or the instruments (e.g., checklists) they use, are *valid* measures of the client's current functioning. Such a concern with a measure's validity is in essence an attempt to establish whether the measure truly does describe or assess what it purports to evaluate. For example, concluding that an individual is an "unfit, abusive" parent because he/she informed the interviewer that spanking was used as a discipline technique once in the past, may be of questionable validity. The use of spanking as a controlling technique might certainly reflect one of the characteristics of an abusive parent. Yet it is only one of many indicators that need to be present. Similarly, concluding that someone has an inferior intelligence because he/she reports withdrawing from school at the age of twelve, fails to consider the entire range of reasons for such a withdrawal. In fact, the question of school attendance does not always attest to one's "ability for schooling." Instead, it may reflect personal interest, health, family conditions, or financial conditions during the school years. So to use the question of "when did you leave school?" as a tool to measure "intelligence" might well be simplistic and invalid.

Another consideration for all individuals employing psychological testing is the degree to which the instruments used are *reliable*. A reliable measure is one that provides relatively consistent results. When human service workers employ checklist items, interview questions, or observational measures, they need to appreciate how these assessment techniques are reactive to varied factors. Such variables might include time of day, client situational state (e.g., hungry, tired), setting (e.g., classroom, office, or home), or even tester conditions (e.g., how the tester is feeling on a particular day). Due to these factors the data collected may turn out to be highly inconsistent. Such inconsistency would then be a reflection of the poor reliability of the instrument used rather than changes within the individual or between the individual and other people or circumstances.

Since human service workers are often the persons making initial contact with clients, the issues of validity and reliability of "testing" tools are especially important. Accordingly, human service workers need to question whether or not the tools they use are in fact measuring what they say they are with consistent results. If not, serious consideration needs to be given to the modification of these invalid and unreliable interview questions, checklists, or observational strategies.

Therefore, in addition to understanding and applying the components of "good" testing (i.e., validity/reliability) to their own interview and observational processes, human service workers need to be better informed about the subtleties of psychological testing, since there appears to be a trend toward an increased use of these workers as psychological testing technicians. There is an increasing demand for B.A./B.S. level personnel who have a human behavior background, and these positions offer preservice training in test administration and scoring.

Also, associate professionals are frequently in a position to provide informal support by assisting in test administration. For example, in the psychiatric wing of a general hospital, the staff practical nurse or mental health technologist may administer a Bender Gestalt Test or Minnesota Multiphasic Personality Inventory (MMPI) to aid the psychologist in the screening section of the intake evaluation.

Training in delivery of services in psychological testing administration and scoring is usually straightforward and does not require a great deal of time or effort. And as many clinical psychologists are finding, human service workers, because of their previous training and experience, may observe and report essential information that might be missed by others. While the psychologist remains the expert in personality and intelligence testing, the allied professional involved in human services can be of great assistance in the areas of referral, administration, and scoring.

This last point is especially important in light of the contemporary use of psychological testing. The value of psychological tests and their results, which during the early years following World War II were viewed as the "absolute answer," are now viewed much more tentatively. Most professionals employ psychological tests as microexperiments, in which the test *samples* the client's attitudes, beliefs, feelings, or behaviors. From this sampling, the mental health worker attempts to generalize a diagnosis regarding the client's state or condition. To remove testing from its once impervious, unquestioned perch and to place it within the framework of a "sampling" tool provides a number of new concerns for those employing such tests.

As with any sample or microexperiment, the value of testing lies in its ability to generalize the data acquired through such sampling to the entire range of client behaviors. Such generalization, however, is often limited by: (1) the narrowness of any one measure used; (2) the setting employed (the psychologist's office, hospital ward, etc.); or (3) the person doing the testing (male, female, black, white, etc.). The inclusion of the human service specialist as an additional source of data collection expands the generalizability of the data collected. By including a variety of testers, settings, and instruments, one can be assured that the data so collected reflect the unique needs and resources of the client and are not simply an artifact of the testing condition.

Another reason for acquiring an understanding about psychological testing lies in the fact that the human service worker often may be in the best position to recommend a *referral* for further testing.

By virtue of their roles, assistant caseworkers, nursing personnel, mental health counselors, hospital technologists, psychiatric workers, and other line personnel have closer contact with people being served by a human service system than psychologists or psychiatrists. In fact, some people who could benefit from a psychological testing evaluation might never receive it if a referral is not made for testing or a therapeutic evaluation by a psychologist. Accordingly, some familiarity with the psychological testing process will help the worker to determine when the client's situation seems likely to benefit from such an action and to facilitate a referral.

The Testing Evaluation Procedure

The psychological testing process involves several steps:

1. The psychologist reviews referral information and purpose of testing.

2. A determination is made whether testing is indicated.
3. If evaluation seems warranted, a group (battery) of tests is chosen.
4. Tests are administered, scored, and interpreted.
5. A report is prepared.

One of the functions of the psychologist is to determine from the referral information and request for testing whether testing is desirable or necessary. *Every refrerral does not necessarily result in testing.*

Not only is psychological evaluation costly and time consuming, but it is also an invasion of a client's privacy. The current consumer movement emphasizes patients' rights to privacy and the importance of professional accountability. Therefore, rather than employing a barrage or shotgun

Table 3.1. Referral Purposes of Psychological Testing

1. *Differential Diagnosis*

Diagnosis sometimes cannot be established by an interview. Observable symptoms may be few, or their meanings may be unclear; symptoms vary from person to person and do not always relate to a single etiology or cause. In such instances, testing is often used to determine how serious and pervasive various problems may be, to elucidate etiology, to differentiate between two similar diagnostic classifications for the client, or to provide *early* clues to the presence of a developing major psychological disorder.

2. *Psychotherapy*

Psychological tests can provide information on a client's personality assets and weak areas, capabilities and difficulties in interpersonal relations, ability to maintain contact with reality, defensive styles, motivations, conflicts, or the possibility of organic involvement. Tests can help the therapist to decide whether to treat the patient with a particular type of therapy. For example, psychoanalysis is not an appropriate technique to use with many types of clients, but testing can help one to decide whether it would be an effective method in particular cases.

3. *Intellectual Assessment*

a.   To determine the presence or absence of organic involvement, the psychosocial factors involved, and the current deficiencies in cases in which a learning disorder is reported.

b.   To establish an intelligence quotient in instances of mental retardation.

c.   To delineate an individual's intellectual strengths and weaknesses.

d.   To assess effects of brain damage.

4. *Vocational/Educational*

a.   To establish current educational achievement (ability) and aptitude (potentiality) levels.

b.   To indicate possible occupational interest areas.

5. *Dangerousness*

a.   To assess homicidal and acting-out potential.

b.   To evaluate suicidal ideation and potential.

approach to testing, one needs to take care to screen out requests for assessment when an interview is all that is needed to obtain the information sought. Along this line, psychologists now try to determine whether the purpose of the evaluation can, in fact, be achieved by testing (see table 3.1). In addition, there is special sensitivity to the need to ensure the protection of the client's right to privacy by selecting and using only those test instruments that are designed for the questions under consideration.

The human service worker can play an essential role in this test-evaluation process. The completeness, clarity, and specificity provided by the worker in the request for testing not only serves to filter out unnecessary assessments, but also assists psychologists in their attempt to focus upon the specific areas to be assessed.

Making a Referral

In the formal sense, referrals are typically made to a psychologist by a medical doctor or agency director. However, in reality it is often a member of the nursing staff, an allied health professional, or a human service worker who informally initiates the process. The proximity of these individuals in the hospital, school, or community to the client enables them to see more readily that additional data are needed before a treatment or management decision can be made concerning the client. In situations in which there is confusion regarding the cause, possibility of organic involvement, or pervasiveness of interpersonal difficulties, the close interaction of these staff members with clients may expose problems that are otherwise unnoticed. The problem might be a learning disorder, personality problem, identity crisis, developmental lag, or visual-motor dysfunction that has gone undetected. In such cases, referrals for testing will be suggested by the health professional, who may also be required to prepare an outline for referral.

When writing a referral for psychological testing, many elements may be included in order to provide an extensive background report. Though in many cases little material is provided the psychologist, the following data are included in most reports:

1. Identifying data.
   Name, address, age, sex, occupation.
2. Reason for referral.
   Illustrations: (a) physician wants to prescribe psychotropic drug for patient who is depressed or frequently anxious, but wants to ensure problem is only situational or minor; (b) psychiatrist is considering taking individual into therapy, but wants to see if patient has enough personal strength and a sufficiently developed self-concept to undergo

insight therapy; (c) school counselor wants to determine if child with a learning disorder is not functioning because of some organic involvement, or whether the cause of the problem is psychological and/or social.
3. Information requested.
Illustrations: (a) description of conflicts and stress areas experienced by person referred; (b) possibility of organic involvement; (c) intellectual abilities and disabilities; (d) recommendations for institutionalization or further hospitalization; (e) suggestions regarding further testing or continued therapy; (f) tentative diagnosis and prognosis for recovery.

In being clear in developing a referral, the human service professional is not attempting to tell the psychologists how to do their job. Rather, as indicated earlier, by being more specific and concrete in the *reason for referral*, and being more focused in noting the *information requested*, the human service professional increases the efficiency and responsiveness of the testing process. For this reason the inclusion of behavioral descriptions, anecdotes, client quotations, and even client work products (e.g., tests, papers, drawings, letters, etc.) that can facilitate the psychologist's understanding of the presenting problem is also encouraged.

Selecting a Battery of Tests

If a psychological assessment seems indicated, a test or series of tests will be chosen based on the aims of the evaluation and the knowledge and experience of the psychologist. There are hundreds of tests to choose from, but only a small portion of these are in widespread use (see table 3.2 and 3.3).

Test selection is determined essentially by the purpose of the evaluation. Obviously, if an intellectual assessment is requested, the evaluator would not choose to administer a personality test. For example, in a personality evaluation some psychologists would favor an objective personality test like the MMPI, while others would select a projective device such as the Rorschach.

The former type of device often is a pencil-and-paper test, requiring the client to respond in a limited way to rather direct questions or statements (e.g., I am afraid of the dark.—True/False). On the other hand, projective devices present the client with ambiguous stimuli, such as inkblots or pictures, and require the client to envisage structure or interpretations for the examiner. These responses are interpreted by the examiner in accordance with his or her theory of personality and psychopathology.

It is rare today for a psychologist to use only one test when conducting an evaluation. Whether the purpose is to determine the client's current level of intellectual functioning or to elucidate some personality dynamics, the

Table 3.2. Widely Used Intelligence Tests

---

1. *Wechsler Adult Intelligence Scale (WAIS). (Wechsler Intelligence Scale for Children (WISC) is the form used for children ages 6 to 16.)*
This psychometric device is one of the most widely utilized individual intelligence tests. It provides information about a person's overall verbal and performance skills. Its subtests also yield measures of the examinee's fund of general information, social comprehension and alertness, ability to abstract and conceptualize, visual-motor skills, auditory recall, as well as a number of other factors contributing to general intelligence.
The WAIS is often reviewed for what it can tell about a person's personality and reality contact. It may be used as part of a test battery along with the Bender Gestalt Test, Rorschach, Thematic Apperception Test, Draw–A Person/House-Tree-Person, and the Sentence Completion Test.
2. *Stanford-Binet Intelligence Scale*
The Stanford-Binet is probably the best known of all individual intelligence tests. Though it has been replaced in the past several years in many settings by the WAIS, it is still in widespread use. It is used with children and adults, and provides, for the most part, information similar to that of the WAIS.
3. *Additional Population Intelligence Tests and Developmental Scales*
   a. *Raven Progressive Matrices.* A group intelligence test for ages 5 to 65.
   b. *Vineland Social Maturity Scale.* A measure of social competence often used with mentally retarded individuals.
   c. *Gesell Developmental Scale.* Scale used to study preschool children's mental growth.
   d. *Shipley Hartford Scale.* Compares vocabulary and abstracting ability as a method of measuring intellectual impairment.
   e. *Peabody Picture Vocabulary Test.* An easily administered test in which the tester can evaluate the examinee's word recognition without the necessity of a verbal response.

---

goal of achieving valid, reliable results dictates that several test devices be employed.

The inner working of one's psyche is currently viewed as only *one* source of a person's behavior. The special demands placed on people by the particular tasks in which they are engaged (e.g., being a parent, teacher, student) and the particular setting in which they operate (e.g., school, home, workplace) are also deemed important today. This shift in focus away from a strictly clinical, "disease within" orientation toward a more community-based, extrapersonal, and interactional model has forced evaluators to increase the use of environmental and behavioral scales as part of their test battery.

The use of these new behavioral tools has created a demand for the development of systematic observational skills. Human service workers, regardless of whether they are involved with administering psychological

Table 3.3. Popular Projective and Objective Personality Tests

1. *Rorschach Inkblot Test*

    One of the most famous projective techniques ever developed, the Rorschach consists of the presentation of ten standardized inkblots for the purpose of eliciting *associations*. These associations are then interpreted.

    There are other inkblot tests (Harrower Inkblot Technique, Holtzman Inkblot Technique), but the Rorschach is by far the most popular. It is used with both children and adults.

2. *Thematic Apperception Technique (TAT)*. *Children's Apperception Technique (CAT) is a similar technique to the TAT, but it was developed (standardized) especially for children.*

    In this projective personality technique, the client is asked to tell a story in response to each picture presented. While this test is comprised of twenty pictures, the psychologist selects only a portion for presentation (some pictures are designed specifically for man or woman, boy or girl). One adaptation of this test is the Blacky Test, in which cartoons are used in place of pictures to elicit stories.

3. *Bender (Visual Motor) Gestalt Test (BGT/BVMGT)*

    This test is used both as a graphomotor technique to help determine the presence of brain damage and as a projective technique from which interpretations about personality makeup are derived. It involves the presentation of nine geometric figures that the client must copy on a piece of paper. In some cases, the administrator may also request the client to recall the figures on paper or to make associations after the copy phase has been completed.

4. *Draw–A Person Test (DAP)*

    In this test, the subject is asked to draw a person and then to draw another person of the opposite sex to the first. This technique is a projective device designed to see how the person projects a body image. A variation of the technique is the House-Tree-Person (HTP).

5. *Minnesota Multiphasic Personality Inventory (MMPI)*

    The best known of the objective, pencil-and-paper personality tests is the MMPI. It comes in three forms: group, individual, and short. The subject is presented with a lengthy questionnaire and asked to respond in a true/false fashion. The MMPI includes both validity scales to check for cheating, malingering, and so on, and a number of clinical scales to measure personality traits and psychopathology.

6. *Other Population Objective Personality Tests*
    a. California Personality Inventory (CPI)
    b. Edwards Personal Preference Schedule (EPPS)
    c. Cattell 16 Personality Factor Questionnaire (16 PF)
    d. Eysenck Personality Inventory (EPI)
    e. Personality Inventory (Bernreuter)

tests or conducting an intake interview, can benefit from sharpening and systematizing such observational abilities. Specifically, there is a need to develop an ability to define, record, and validate their behavioral observations.

Human service workers need to begin to identify specific *actions* upon which to center their attention during interviews or screenings. Simply saying that one is observing the person for signs of being "bad" or "disturbed" does not lend to valid, reliable observation. However, *operationally defining* "bad" as "every time the client punches the interviewer," or "disturbed" as "each time the client deliberately bites him/herself," will provide the needed concrete, countable, behavioral referrent for ensuring valid, reliable observation.

The worker also needs to develop or employ tools that will facilitate the measurement and recording of these bahaviors. Often mechanical devices such as a simple golf stroke counter can assist in recording the frequency with which the observed behavior has occurred. Such frequency counts will assist the worker in drawing conclusions about the increase or decrease of the behavior under a variety of conditions or settings. Finally, in an attempt to increase the accuracy of their observation, human service workers need to validate their observations by contrasting their findings with those obtained from other instruments or observers.

As can be seen, becoming a trained, systematic observer, while not being easy, is an essential ingredient to the work of the human service professional.

Administration, Scoring, and Interpretation

The testing and evaluation procedure may stretch over several hours or several days, depending on such factors as tests used, experience of the clinician, and type of individual being evaluated.

A clinician familiar with a particular test battery may be able to complete a personality evaluation of a moderately depressed, slightly confused individual in a matter of hours. Conversely, a psychology intern assigned to evaluate a deeply disturbed individual may have to extend the testing over a period of days because of the client's poor attention span. Or a novice practitioner might have to spend long hours developing subtle interpretations from the material gleaned during the session.

Interpretation—particularly in the case of projective tests—requires a great deal of effort from any psychologist. It is the heart of the evaluation process. Unless one has a thorough knowledge of human development and of psychopathology, and a coherent theory of personality organization, much can be lost in the interpretation procedure. This is why the key tasks of interpretation and report preparation are the province of the psychologist.

The Psychological Report

Once the evaluation is completed, a report is prepared for the professional (physician, psychiatrist, teacher) or agency (clinic, hospital, school) that made the referral. The wording and style of the report are more or less technical, depending on the recipient's needs and professional status. Since the purpose of psychological testing is to facilitate decision making, the report reflecting the data upon which such decisions are to be based needs to be presented in *clear, understandable* language. The use of professional jargon such as "ego alien," "ego syntonic," "cognitive distortions," etc., often prove to be an efficient way of conveying information among similarly trained professionals. However, reports are often presented to varied readership and as such an overreliance on such professional jargon might prove confusing and distracting. Behavioral descriptions, verbatim reporting, and concrete examples designed to assist the reader to fully understand the data presented are often more profitable. In addition, though a good deal of data about the client has been gathered during the evaluation, the bulk of the report will center on the key questions asked in the referral.

While clinical psychologists vary in their choices of format for the report, the following information is typical of the content of a normal evaluation:

1. Identifying data
2. Appearance of subject during testing
3. Test-taking behavior
4. Intellectual assessment
5. Personality functioning
6. Psychological/organic problems (psychopathology)
7. Diagnosis
8. Prognosis
9. Summary and conclusions
10. Recommendations

Today, laws in most states permit the client to have access to psychological reports. This point further supports the need to avoid jargon when writing a report. In addition, the fact that a client may desire access and feedback regarding the test results necessitates that the referring agent be prepared to interpret the test data meaningfully. The report writer, therefore, should be encouraged to follow up on the report, in order to clarify any points of confusion that may arise for the human service worker or the person being assessed.

Summary

Psychological testing involves a number of steps. Though this process is conducted by, or under the supervision of, a clinical psychologist, the human service worker often plays an important part. Situations in which psychological testing seems indicated are often observed and reported by nursing personnel, allied health professionals, and human service workers. Though in many systems these individuals may not be in positions to make direct referrals, they are often responsible for advising their administrator when such referrals appear to be appropriate.

Assistant caseworkers, for example, might note that intelligence and vocational interest questionnaires would provide helpful information to certain clients who are having problems making occupational adjustments or choices; a physician's associate might observe that the personality problems of the patient the general physician is treating with antidepressants are more extensive than appears on the surface; and a teacher might be confused about the cause and implications of a learning disability in one of his or her quiet students. If referral is not made or the problem not brought to the attention of an employer, needed psychological testing may not be undertaken in time to avert more serious problems.

Allied health personnel may often administer some forms of psychological testing devices under the supervision of a clinician. Psychological testing technicians are growing in number. Associate mental health professionals are becoming involved as members of psychological testing teams, just as physical health personnel are working with medical professionals.

Whatever the role of the worker or professional, whether in medical, psychological, educational, or social services, basic familiarity with the process of psychological testing is required. Only when line health personnel appreciate the function of psychological testing, can it be expected that its use will be extended to all who may benefit from it.

nosology

problem definition

4 / *diagnostic classification*

As human service professionals, trained to be empathic and respecting of the human conditions, we are generally appalled by the practices of stereotyping and "pigeonholing" people. Yet, though one might argue that labels are normally too general and impersonal for people, as helpers we often still see the process of diagnostic labeling as a viable and valuable practice. In this area, medicine's long-term use of categorization has often served as the prototype to be followed.

Medicine employs diagnosis and classification as an essential element in the care and treatment of patients. The very concept of diagnosis often conjures up images of stethoscopes, needles, blood/urine analyses, and the ponderous look of the physician weighing the various data reflecting a patient's condition. This is not surprising, for medicine has found the diagnostic-classification process a means for structuring great masses of information into meaningful and manageable units. However, the usefulness of this process within the mental health arena is still under question. In medicine, as with other branches of science, the purpose of a taxonomy or classification system is to provide order and direction to what first appears to be a host of unrelated diverse phenomena. The diagnostic classification process used in medicine is much more than a mere process of labeling. It is a process that is indispensable to the prescription and treatment of the person under one's care.

The process begins by a consideration of the presenting complaint and overt symptoms. The physician notes a patient's blood pressure, temperature, and verbalized aches and pains, and thus begins the diagnostic-classification process. However, since one's blood pressure, temperature, or pain may be a reflection of a number of underlying problems, additional diagnostic information will be gathered (e.g., blood and urine analyses, x-ray). Once all of the data have been compiled, the physician then attempts to identify the unique pattern of symptoms evidenced. The identification of this syndrome (symptom pattern) facilitates the physician's understanding of the possible underlying causes for the disorder (etiology), as well as its predictive course or outcome (prognosis) and preferred method of treatment. Further, noting the existence of this or that unique and distinct syndrome enables practitioners to easily and accurately communicate information among themselves. In addition, such identification assists researchers to pursue in-depth understanding of the disorder in question.

Because of mental health's historical affiliation with medicine and the promotion of the medical model of mental illness (see introduction), it was natural that similar taxonomies would be developed for mental disorders. Views as to the value of these taxonomies and the process of classification as applied within the mental health arena have been quite varied. Many human service professionals suggest that the use of a label or a classification is fraught with a number of potential pitfalls. It is argued that labeling leads people to assume things about those who are labeled that are in fact not true. Labels may also tend to inappropriately and simplistically categorize an individual in an overly generalized way, without adequately representing the unique human condition of that individual.

Even with the aforementioned limitations, however, diagnostic labels can be useful. If used properly, they can prove to be efficient ways of communication among professionals. Categorizing this versus that as "edible" or "inedible," for instance, saves an individual much time and energy from the task of tasting and experimenting with each food item. Similarly, identifying one organism as part of this phylum or that class provides the researcher with clear guidelines for understanding the nature of the organism, its predictable patterns, and its relationship with others within this and other phyla or classes.

In medicine and mental health services, a special form of classification is used for the identification of pathological conditions. Taxonomies of pathological conditions are termed "nosologies." Nosologies attempt to cluster *symptoms* (i.e., behavioral descriptions/manifestations of one's feelings, thinking, or actions) into *syndromes* (i.e., a distinct, correlated set of symptoms). For example, let us assume that an individual is presented to the psychologist with the following symptoms: loss of appetite; reduction in energy or desire to do anything; experience of suicidal thoughts and feelings of reprisal; frequent excessive crying and feelings of hopelessness. The psychologist may find that the *behavioral* (inability to perform previously successful tasks); *emotional* (feelings of sadness, discouragement); and *cognitive* (sense of personal worthlessness and hopelessness) symptoms cluster together into a depressive syndrome.

Employing the label of "depression" provides an economical means for communicating the aforementioned symptoms. However, as previously suggested, nosological systems and diagnostic labels are intended to do more than simply provide shorthand notation for lists of symptoms.

Nosologies also establish that each syndrome is distinct, with unique etiology (cause), prognosis (predictive course and outcome), and preferred treatment regimen. In medicine, for example, the diagnosis of acute appendicitis not only implies a cluster of symptoms (e.g., fever, abdominal distress, nausea), but also etiology (damaged or diseased appendix) and prescribed treatment (operation). Similarly, the human service worker presented with a child manifesting slow or retarded development, an unusually strong and distinctive odor, physical uncoordination, and evidence of intellectual retardation may "cluster" these symptoms into a pattern reflective of the PKU syndrome. PKU or phenylketonuria is a genetic disorder that makes it impossible for a child to metabolize phenylalanine (i.e., a protein substance found in many foods). The accumulation of this substance in the child's system creates the aforementioned symptoms. Thus, detecting the PKU syndrome assists the human service worker to understand the etiology (genetic defect and phenylalanine buildup); prognosis (irreversible brain damage unless intervention occurs); and prescribed treatment (special low phenylalanine diet and remedial education).

While there are numerous examples of the potential value of such categorization and diagnostic labels, their usefulness is limited by the validity of the classification system that they reflect. Thus, although the human service profession employs a system of classification for the categorization of mental and behavioral disturbances, the validity of this system and its basic value has been an issue of much discussion and remains so today.

Early Classification Efforts

As noted in the introduction, the human service profession moved from a period of demonology, in which all mental disorders were "classified" as symptomatic of possession, to an era of enlightenment, in which mental illness was viewed as that—a human illness. In moving away from these early days of trephining and bloodletting, those treating the mentally ill soon came to recognize the existence of different illnesses and, therefore, the need for different treatments. During the late nineteenth century and early twentieth century a number of nosological systems were established.

Emil Kraepelin (1856–1926), a German psychiatrist, is generally credited with developing the first systematic and widely accepted classification schema for mental disorders. Kraepelin viewed mental disorders as "diseases" that originated in some biological-metabolical defect. He compiled thousands of case histories. Sorting the cases, Kraepelin noted that they reflected not mere random symptoms, but relatively consistent patterns, or groupings. Upon this observation Kraepelin began the process of identifying separate "diagnostic syndromes" and with them, the first diagnostic-classification system of mental illness.

Kraepelin defined and classified two major forms of severe mental illness. The first and statistically most prevalent syndrome was what he termed "dementia praecox." The disorder was described as having an onset early in one's life (i.e., *praecox*) and generally progressed to an incurable and apparently irreversible madness (i.e., *dementia*). What Kraepelin was describing has since been labeled "schizophrenia." The second category identified by Kraepelin was "manic-depressive psychosis." Kraepelin noted that this syndrome generally consisted of extreme states of elation and excitement (i.e., *mania*) and melancholia (i.e., *depression*), which often occurred in cyclic fashion.

Following upon Kraepelin's work a number of efforts were made to develop the *definitive* classification system. In 1917, the Committee on Statistics of the American Psychiatric Association (APA) adopted a standard nomenclature. In 1939, the World Health Organization (WHO) added mental disorders to their International List of Causes of Death, and so the proliferation of classification systems began.

The variety of classifications emerging impeded, rather than facilitated, communication within the profession; and, as such, numerous attempts were made at developing a more coherent, generally accepted system. Both the World Organization and the American Psychiatric Association continued modifying their systems in an attempt to develop a coordinated, comprehensive classification system.

In 1968, the American Psychiatric Association developed its second version of the *Diagnostic and Statistical Manual* (DSM II). The system developed by the APA was closely in line with that produced in the 1969 revision of the World Health Organization's system of classification. While many of the labels employed were similar, diagnostic criteria and descriptions still varied.

Criticism of the Classification Model

The struggle to find a unified system and the problems stemming from the utilization of two such similar, yet clearly distinct systems as those produced by the APA and the WHO began to stimulate criticism of the use of classification systems.

Classification as Unreliable.   One principal line of criticism aired against the use of a diagnostic classification system is that the systems so far created have proved to be *unreliable*. Critics following this line of argument note that symptoms attributed to one diagnostic category overlap and are found often in other categories as well. Because of this overlap, the assignment of labels to a cluster of symptoms proves quite inconsistent (i.e., unreliable). Further, since clients often show a variety of symptoms, they do not easily "fit" into any one diagnostic category. The clinician is forced to make a judgment regarding the primary symptom profile and the accompanying diagnostic label. Such a judgment is often affected by the clinician's theoretical orientation (behavioral, humanistic, psychoanalytic, etc.). Further, judgment and subsequent classification can be affected by nonrelevant or nonclinical characteristics of the patient (e.g., social status, sex, race).

Since a primary value of a diagnostic, nosological system is to facilitate communication among professionals, such unreliability appears to fly in the face of the proposed value. If one is to communicate knowledge about a specific disorder, then one must be sure that the label applied to this disorder is *consistently* understood to represent that *one* symptom formation. Even when agreement regarding diagnosis is established, there is rarely agreement among clinicians regarding etiology or prescribed mode of treatment. These factors (i.e., etiology and treatment regimen) appear dictated by one's professional training or theoretical model, and not the diagnostic syndrome under investigation.

Classification as Invalid. While many critics point to the difficulty of finding agreement or consistency in the labels applied, others question the very *validity* of such diagnostic labels.

Thomas Szasz (1960) argues that mental illness is a social myth. Szasz posits that what has been labeled as "mental illness" is nothing more than *unsolved problems of living.* As such, the question being raised is whether or not "mental illness" as a category or entity even exists.

For example, does saying that a person is experiencing a sense of global fear or anxiety imply that he is ill? Is an individual who experiences extended and debilitating periods of melancholy also providing evidence of the existence of a "disease?" Furthermore, critics of the classification system inquire, "How can it be that such diagnosis, which supposedly reflects the existence of a real disease or illness, is founded on so many dissimilar, inconsistent criteria?" Or, "How can it be that a disease can be eradicated through social-political pressure or by simply changing a definition, as was the case when the American Psychiatric Association *removed* homosexuality from its list of sexual deviances?" These and other similar questions are raised by professionals who are attacking the basic validity of classification and nosologies for the human services.

Classification as Dehumanizing. Finally, as an extension of the abovementioned criticisms (i.e., unreliable and invalid), many critics point to the basic injustice and dehumanization of the labeling process. The process of assigning a label, it is argued, is both stigmatizing and dehumanizing. Labeling a client or patient creates a condition in which an individual with a "problem of living" is victimized by the mental health profession. Terms such as "mental illness," "neurosis," and "psychosis," not only stigmatize people, but may in fact lead to development of the symptoms they supposedly describe. Calling a person "crazy" or "mentally ill" oftentimes creates a condition in which he/she is shunned, mistreated, ridiculed, and forced into deviant forms of behavior.

Much has been written about the self-fulfilling prophecy. That is, if one is told, often enough, that he/she *is* a certain way, he/she tends to behave in ways that confirm this prophecy. Thus, it may be suggested that by labeling a person as "deviant," the identification and labeling itself promotes the development of the deviant symptoms. The question then becomes, "Are we merely diagnosing and describing an existing condition, or are we in fact creating the condition through this diagnostic process?" Further, it is argued that labeling dehumanizes an individual. Diagnostic labels foster a situation in which the person is treated as a "syndrome" (e.g., "the depressed client in room 18" or "the psychotic in ward B") rather than as a human being with a variety of individual potentials and resources.

Many of those criticizing the previous attempts at classification have called for the abandonment of such diagnostic-classification practices. However, rather than discarding diagnostic classification (which might prove to be a case of throwing the baby out with the bath water), consideration needs to be given to rectifying the specific weaknesses of the previous efforts.

DSM III—Attempting to "Right" the "Wrongs"

In 1980, the American Psychiatric Association published its third edition of the *Diagnostic and Statistical Manual of Mental Disorders* (DSM III). The DSM III is a broadly based and eclectic classification system that was created in response to the criticism raised about the previous systems.

The goal of the task force developing the manual was to provide a clinically useful, reliable set of diagnostic categories. DSM III, therefore, differs from its predecessors in that (1) it provides extensive *operational definitions* and behavioral descriptions of the essential and associated features of each syndrome; (2) details specific *diagnostic criteria* to guide decision making regarding the assignment of a diagnosis; and (3) promotes the use of a holistic orientation in the classification of mental disorder. This final point is aided by the manual's use of a *multiaxial* classification process.

Operational Definitions. In response to the concerns about reliability of classification, the authors of the DSM III have provided extensive behavioral descriptions of the symptomatology involved in each syndrome. The manual provides description of both the "essential" and "associated" features of the syndrome (see table 4.1). In order to further depict the distinct nature of each syndrome, these descriptions are followed by information regarding expected age of onset, course of development, degree of impairment, complications, prevalence, sex ratios, and expected family patterns.

Diagnostic Criteria. In order to increase the precision and consistency of diagnostic procedures, DSM III provides specific diagnostic criteria to be employed prior to assigning a diagnostic label. These criteria involve the appearance of specific symptoms, frequency and duration guidelines, age of onset guidelines, and delimiters or restrictions (see table 4.2).

Multiaxial Process. A major innovation of the DSM III is its use of a multidimensional or multiaxial approach to the diagnostic process. The use of a multiaxial format forces the clinician out of a single bias or narrow theoretical perspective and promotes the use of a broad range of information as the basis for making diagnostic decisions.

The DSM III provides five dimensions or "axes" upon which to classify a particular syndrome. Axes I and II contain the official diagnostic categories of all mental disorders (see tables 4.3 and 4.4).

Axis III points to the client's current physical condition, which may be potentially relevant to the understanding and management of the problem under investigation. Axis IV provides a system for assessing the psychosocial stressors active in the client's life, and Axis V identifies the client's highest level of adaptive functioning during the past year (see table 4.5).

Table 4.1. Example of Behavioral Description of Generalized Anxiety Disorder*

The essential feature is generalized, persistent anxiety of at least one month's duration. . . .

Although the specific manifestations of anxiety vary from individual to individual, generally there are signs of motor tension, autonomic hyperactivity, apprehensive expectations, and vigilance and scanning.

Associated Features. Mild depressive symptoms are common.

Impairment. Impairment in social or occupational functioning is rarely more than mild.

Complications. Abuse of alcohol, barbiturates, and antianxiety medications is common.

Age at onset, course, predisposing factors, prevalence, sex ratio, and familial patterns. No information.

Differential Diagnosis. Physical disorders such as Hyperthyroidism and Organic Mental Disorders, such as Caffeine Intoxication, must be ruled out.

---

* From the *Diagnostic and Statistical Manual of Mental Disorders (DSM III)* by the American Psychiatric Association. Copyright 1980 the American Psychiatric Association. Reprinted by permission.

Table 4.2. Diagnostic Criteria for Generalized Anxiety Disorder*

A. Generalized, persistent anxiety is manifested by symptoms from three of the following four categories:

   (1) *Motor tension.* Shakiness, jitteriness, jumpiness, trembling, tension, muscle aches, fatigability, and inability to relax are common complaints.

   (2) *Autonomic hyperactivity.* There may be sweating, heart pounding or racing, cold, clammy hands, dry mouth, dizziness, light-headedness, paresthesias (tingling in hands and feet), upset stomach, hot or cold spells, frequent urination, diarrhea, discomfort in the pit of the stomach, lump in the throat, flushing, pallor, and high resting pulse and respiration rate.

   (3) *Apprehensive expectation.* The individual is generally apprehensive and continually feels anxious, worries, ruminates, and anticipates that something bad will happen to himself or herself (e.g., fear of fainting, losing control, dying) or others.

   (4) *Vigilance and Scanning.* Apprehensive expectation may cause hyper-attentiveness so that the individual feels "on edge," impatient, or irritable. There may be complaints of distractibility, difficulty in concentrating, insomnia, difficulty falling asleep, interrupted sleep, and fatigue on awakening.

B. The anxious mood has been continuous for at least one month.

C. Not due to another mental disorder, such as a Depressive Disorder or Schizophrenia.

D. At least 18 years of age.

Table 4.3. Axis I: Clinical Syndromes Listed in DSM III (1980)

Disorders Usually First Evident in Infancy, Childhood, or Adolescence

Organic Mental Disorders	Somatoform Disorders
Substance Use Disorders	Dissociative Disorders
Schizophrenic Disorders	Psychosexual Disorders
Paranoid Disorders	Psychological Factors Affecting
Affective Disorders	Physical Condition
Anxiety Disorders	

Table 4.4. Axis II: Personality Disorders and Specific Developmental Disorders Listed in DSM III (1980)

Personality Disorders
   paranoid, schizoid, schizotypal, histrionic, narcissistic, antisocial, borderline, avoidant, dependent, compulsive, passive-aggressive

Specific Developmental Disorders
   reading, arithmetic, language, articulation

---

* Tables 4.2, 4.3, 4.4, and 4.5 are from the *Diagnostic and Statistical Manual of Mental Disorders (DSM III)* by the American Psychiatric Association. Copyright 1980 the American Psychiatric Association. Reprinted by permission.

Table 4.5. Axes III, IV, V of the DSM III (1980)

AXIS III: Physical Disorders or Conditions

Permits the clinician to indicate any current physical disorder or condition that is potentially relevant to the understanding or management of the individual. These are the conditions outside of the mental disorders section ICD–9–CM (APA, 1980, p. 26).

AXIS IV: Ratings of Severity of Psychosocial Stressors

1. none
2. minimal (e.g., minor violation of law)
3. mild (e.g., argument with neighbor)
4. moderate (e.g., death of close friend)
5. severe (e.g., serious personal illness)
6. extreme (e.g., death of close relative)
7. catastrophic (e.g., natural disaster)

AXIS V: Highest Level of Adaptive Functioning Past Year

1. superior: unusually effective in social relations, occupation, and use of leisure time (e.g., single parent in reduced circumstances takes excellent care of children, has warm friendships and a hobby)
2. very good: better than average in job, leisure time, and social functioning (e.g., retired person does volunteer work, sees old friends)
3. good: no more than slight impairment in either occupational or social functioning (e.g., individual with many friends does a difficult job extremely well, but finds it a strain)
4. fair: moderate impairment in either social or occupational functioning or some impairment in both (e.g., lawyer has trouble carrying through assignments, has almost no close friends)
5. poor: marked impairment in either social or occupational functioning or moderate impairment in both (e.g., man with one or two friends has trouble holding a job for more than a few weeks)
6. very poor: marked impairment in social and occupational functioning (e.g., woman is unable to do any housework and has violent outbursts)
7. grossly impaired: gross impairment in virtually all areas of functioning (e.g., elderly man needs supervision in maintaining personal hygiene, is usually incoherent)

Even though the DSM III falls short of being *the* definitive classification system, it can be justifiably praised for its assets. Research has demonstrated that its specificity of diagnostic criteria and use of behavioral description has increased the reliability of the diagnostic process. Further, its promotion of a holistic, multitheoretical approach certainly adds to the comprehensiveness of the system. But perhaps the ultimate test of any such system rests in the value it holds for those who serve people in need.

Summary

The current chapter has presented a definition of nosology and attempted to outline the proposed value of classifications system to the diagnostic process. While earlier attempts at developing such systems for the classification of mental disorders have been fraught with problems, the solution is not to abandon these efforts, but to attempt to rectify the previous shortcomings.

Previous diagnostic classification systems have proven to be unreliable (i.e., providing inconsistent diagnosis) and have often led to stigmatizing those so labeled. In 1980, the American Psychiatric Association completed its third revision of the *Diagnostic and Statistical Manual of Mental Disorders* (DMS III). The manual attempts to improve the validity and reliability of the diagnostic process by (1) employing extensive behavioral descriptions of each syndrome listed; (2) providing a clear listing of diagnostic criteria for each diagnosis; and (3) promoting a multidimensional or multiaxial approach to the diagnostic process.

The authors of the DSM III, and the early research efforts based on it, have demonstrated that it has ameliorated many of the shortcomings of previous classification systems. Its ultimate value to the human service professional is still waiting to be established.

5 / anxiety

It can be said that anxiety is essential for the maintaining of one's life. Most individuals experience a degree of tension, apprehension, and anxiety in response to stress. When present at an acceptable degree or functional level, it alerts persons to impending dangers and thus motivates them to appropriate action. If anxiety is absent, dangers may go unrecognized or be ignored, encouraging fatal or amoral risk-taking behavior.

Neurotic anxiety, however, is persistent and exaggerated; also, it is not commensurate with the actual threat of the stressful encounter. Such extreme, inappropriate levels of anxiety will prove debilitating rather than facilitating to one's well-being and protection. In extremes, anxiety may physically immobilize the individual, thus engulfing him or her in the threatening situation that originally triggered the initial anxiety. Furthermore, extreme anxiety proves detrimental to one's psychological well-being and physical survival. It can stimulate extended periods of stress reaction and with it the damaging effects of prolonged muscle tension (e.g., cramps, aches, tremors, fatigue) and autonomic innervation (e.g., ulcers, migraines) and block the rational thinking and problem solving required to adequately cope with the stress at hand. In an extreme situation, acute anxiety reaction can occur and even suicide or homicide might result.

Anxiety is commonly found and must be treated with skill and care. Whether in an exaggerated form, as in an acute anxiety reaction, or more commonly as part of an organically or functionally based pathological syndrome, the human service workers can expect to encounter it in hospital and private practice, and in community health centers.

Symptoms of Anxiety

The DSM III (APA, 1980, p. 225) notes that in the category of *anxiety disorders*, anxiety appears as either the predominant symptom (e.g., in panic disorder, generalized anxiety disorder) or as a result of attempting to master other clinical symptoms (e.g., when confronting a fearful object as in phobic disorder). The attempt to diagnose anxiety states is often complicated by the fact that anxiety may mask itself with a wide variety of symptoms.

There are a number of physical disorders that may appear similar to anxiety reactions. In rare instances, an anxiety attack may be initially mistaken for an acute gallbladder attack. More commonly, a person experiencing extreme anxiety symptoms may be misdiagnosed as suffering from a myocardial infarction. In such instances, the patient may even be admitted to a coronary care unit until laboratory and ECG findings rule out a heart problem. In addition, some individuals may attempt to relieve their anxiety by employment of alcohol and barbiturates and thus be viewed as substance abusers rather than individuals with anxiety disorders.

Consequently, it is important for medical and human service personnel to be able to recognize the symptoms of an anxiety reaction, especially when chemical and neurological tests fail to support the presence of such organic problems as hyperthyroidism or a myocardial infarction.

Diagnostically, the essential feature of an anxiety attack is the recurrent panic (anxiety), which appears suddenly and occurs at times unpredictably. The attack is characterized by intense apprehension, fear or terror, and feelings of impending doom. The diagnostic criteria for an anxiety attack or panic disorder are listed in table 5.1.

Table 5.1. Diagnostic Criteria for Panic Disorder*

A. At least three panic attacks within a three-week period in circumstances other than during marked physical exertion or in a life-threatening situation.

B. Panic attacks are manifested by discrete periods of apprehension or fear, and at least four of the following symptoms appear during each attack:

    (1) dyspnea (difficulty in breathing)
    (2) palpitations
    (3) chest pain or discomfort
    (4) choking or smothering sensations
    (5) dizziness, vertigo, or unsteady feelings
    (6) feelings of unreality
    (7) paresthesias (tingling in hands or feet)
    (8) hot and cold flashes
    (9) sweating
    (10) faintness
    (11) trembling or shaking
    (12) fear of dying, going crazy, or doing something uncontrolled during an attack

C. Not due to a physical disorder or another mental disorder.

D. The disorder is not associated with agoraphobia.

---

* From the *Diagnostic and Statistical Manual of Mental Disorders (DSM III)* by the American Psychiatric Association. Copyright 1980 the American Psychiatric Association. Reprinted by permission.

Often, following such bouts of anxiety, the individual develops a dread of the attacks themselves. Individuals may find that they are experiencing generalized, persistent anxiety. The persistent experience of such anxiety for at least one month's duration may signal the existence of a *generalized anxiety disorder*. The specific description and diagnostic criteria of this syndrome have been previously noted in chapter 4 (see tables 4.1 and 4.2).

It should be noted, however, that these signs may not be clearly present, as in the case of minor episodic anxiety. The worker must also be alert to psychological signs shown by anxious clients and mindful of the fact that they, too, may not become evident until the person is thoroughly questioned and observed.

Statements by the client such as: "I feel extremely nervous and upset," or "Lately I just don't feel well, I'm so jittery," will provide the interviewer with clues to the presence of anxiety. Occasionally it is not so obvious that the person is suffering from anxiety, as when physical symptoms like fatigue or insomnia are described without any reference to anxiety. Or, there may be references to irritability and tension that appear to be normal responses in today's fast-paced society and that the individual may rationalize with such remarks as: "I'm so keyed up I can't relax. I guess I've just been working too hard." Or: "I don't seem as decisive anymore. I used to be a deliberate thinker. Probably the job and the kids are getting to me."

Further questioning may reveal that environmental factors may, in fact, be the cause, and the anxiety can be expected to subside when the pressure is relieved. Since everyone is subject to anxious periods, this is a common occurrence with tense clients. However, if the client's concerns have been so persistent that they require medical or psychological attention, or if the source of the anxiety is masked or hidden, the worker may have cause for concern.

Etiology

There is no single or key cause of anxiety. The reasons for anxiety, like the constellation of overt signs it produces, can vary greatly from individual to individual. Accordingly, investigators should attempt to determine what was happening during those times in the client's life that featured sudden onset or increase in the symptoms of anxiety.

"You say you really feel uptight now. When did you start feeling tense like this?"

"From what you say, I gather you're often quite jittery and that you're normally a pretty nervous person. Well, I wonder if there are times when you're especially anxious; you know, more upset than usual?"

By determining precipitating factors, the anxiety-provoking situation can be examined and the individual reeducated to deal with fears or unrealistic elements, and thus helped to function more normally.

Just as there is no single cause of anxiety, there is no singularly accepted theoretical explanation for anxiety states. The classical, psychodynamic approach generally posits that anxiety falls into one of four categories: *impulse anxiety, separation anxiety, castration anxiety,* or *guilt anxiety.*

Impulse anxiety (id anxiety) stems from infancy and arises when persons experience the vague fear that they will lose control and act asocially or illogically. Separation anxiety arises when there is a threat of interpersonal loss or abandonment. Castration anxiety is related to the early childhood fear of genital mutilation; in an adult it is more generally seen as a fear of any bodily damage. Guilt (superego) anxiety comes about when a person transgresses some established moral principle or law.

More recently, the work of two former psychoanalysts, Albert Ellis and Aaron Beck, has refocused attention from the "unconscious" determinents of anxiety to the identification of the "thoughts" and "beliefs" held by clients during states of anxiety or panic. According to this *cognitive behavioral* perspective, people are disturbed not by the events they experience (e.g., seeing a snake, having to give a speech, or going for a job interview), but rather by the interpretations or beliefs they hold about these events. Thus, anxiety reactions are attributed to the fact that the anxious client viewing these life stressors (e.g., snakes, new job) interpret them, not as mere inconveniences or potential disappointments, but as *absolutely unbearable catastrophes.* Once the life stressor is so identified, the anxious client reacts to the mental interpretation of the event (i.e., unbearable catastrophe), rather than to the actual, objective conditions of the event. Thus from a cognitive-behavioral perspective, anxiety is the result of an individual's faulty perception and cognitive distortions. Specifically, anxious individuals often err in their interpretation by *inaccurately magnifying* the actual threat value of a circumstance, *overgeneralizing* the conditions of threat, *minimizing* their own capabilities of handling the situation, and *projecting* future conditions of doom or catastrophe.

The origin of some types of anxiety-producing behavior can sometimes be uncovered by a psychotherapist when the client's childhood experience is explored. For example, in a case in which guilt anxiety was causing problems for a young man in his twenties when he went on dates, the therapist discovered that the client's mother had repeatedly told him when he was in his teens: "Remember, sex is something dirty. If you do it in marriage I guess it's OK—men can't help enjoying themselves. But to do it outside of marriage is a sin! If you do it with some young lady before you're married to her you will get punished. She might get pregnant, then everyone will be angry and ashamed of you. She might give you venereal disease and then that will make you blind. So don't do anything but give the girls you go out with a brief good-night kiss. If you do anything else, it will lead to something."

When this person grew older he realized that his mother had given him bad advice, but the moral sanction she had established remained. He had incorporated her restrictions early in life—at a time when he needed and depended on her love. Now, beneath his awareness, the early message was producing inner turmoil when he transgressed an unconscious restriction.

Handling Anxiety

Whatever the cause, anxiety produces distress. At the minimum, it is uncomfortable to be anxious, and at the other extreme, it may generate actual panic. To deal with such unpleasant or unbearable feelings, the person may deliberately or unconsciously employ techniques to obtain relief. When these methods are within the person's level of awareness, they are called "coping mechanisms." If they are unconsciously employed, they are termed "defense mechanisms."

Coping Mechanisms. Most of the things people do to handle feelings of uneasiness connected with anxiety involve processes that serve to bind, avoid, or reduce the anxiety.

Since anxiety may be a vague or undefined fear, the person experiencing emotional distress is subject to a general but pervasive feeling of discomfort. That is called "free-floating anxiety" and is a common experience for most people.

In response to this, efforts are usually made to connect the anxious feelings with a particular cause. A typical reaction may be expressed as: "I don't know what's bothering me. If I knew, I would feel better—I could at least handle it a little better."

This searching process is beneficial so long as it does not lead to actual brooding, and it should be encouraged by the worker when dealing with anxious patients.

> *Client:* "I just feel so funny today—like I have butterflies in my stomach."
> *Worker:* "What do you think is causing it?"
> *Ct.:* "That's it, I just don't know. Maybe if I knew, I wouldn't feel so bad."
> *W.:* "Well, possibly it's all the tests you had done here in the hospital. Maybe you're worried about their results and you feel impatient about getting them on the one hand, but afraid to hear what they are going to say on the other."
> *Ct.:* "That's silly to be upset about the tests. I mean, I should be happy that they're being done. At least I'll know then if something is wrong. To be anxious about the tests would be silly on my part."
> *W.:* "I can see what you're saying, Mr. Jones, but I don't think it would be silly for you to be anxious about the results of the tests. Most people are, because in today's society people are not trained to wait for results. With all the

computers, answers seem to spurt out so quickly. Possibly you're a little angry that it takes so long for modern medicine to get the results—particularly when you are so upset and uncomfortable in the hospital. I guess, in essence, I'm saying it's understandable if you're a bit anxious and somewhat angry at having to wait. Everyone who comes in for tests usually feels that way to some degree."

Ct.: "I think I see what you mean. Well, it's just that I don't want to be irritable with the people that are trying to find out if anything is wrong with me, but I am getting jittery and I wish I knew already. . . ."

If the searching process uncovers an unrealistic fear, it can be dealt with. Even if the cause the client ascribes his anxiety to isn't actually related to his underlying fear, temporary relief will usually occur. ("Better the devil you know, than the one you don't.")

Once the anxious person identifies the presumed cause of the problem, coping mechanisms can take the form of avoidance of tension-reduction techniques. If giving a speech produces anxiety, a student may avoid courses or situations in which he or she becomes the center of attention. In the case of a marriage problem, the anxious wife may take barbiturates or drink alcohol to lessen stress. More generally, however, stress is dealt with by conscious suppression—forgetting about thoughts or situations that cause unease or nervousness.

Clearly, there are numerous ways people prevent anxiety from becoming severe. These coping mechanisms are easily exposed and normally do not have nearly as strong an impact on a person's personality as do defense mechanisms.

Defense Mechanisms. The "normal" person has a number of devices that function to deal with any underlying conflicts or drives that threaten to erupt into consciousness and cause anxiety. When these devices fail, the person becomes upset; some awareness of their presence may develop. If the problem persists, leading to extreme dependence on defense mechanisms, a disruptive life style may manifest itself. Subsequently, the individual may be termed "neurotic" or otherwise be classified within the abnormal range. Even if the labeling process is avoided, excessive use of defense mechanisms will be viewed by others as strange or weird behavior.

Though there are many types of defense mechanisms, some have been studied more extensively than others and thus are better known.

1. Repression—unconscious forgetting
2. Projection—assigning of one's own unacceptable impulses to someone else
3. Denial—acting as if some idea, problem, thought, and so on does not exist
4. Reaction formation—acting directly opposite to one's unconscious wishes

5. Rationalization—an unconscious mechanism that produces a justification for one's overt behavior
6. Displacement—the redirection of attention or emotion from one person or object to a more acceptable one

Certain defense mechanisms have particular import for allied health personnel since they are directly related to patient care. One of these is *regression*, in which there is a return to a previous developmental level in which emotional gratification was assured. This may occur when an individual is admitted to the hospital and put in a dependency position during a stressful period of illness, causing infantile forms of behavior to surface.

Faced with the anxiety of surgery and confinement to bed in a hospital gown, even a middle-aged female executive may behave like a little girl. Rather than reacting in a mature and responsible manner, she may become demanding, emotional, and surprisingly stubborn.

In a similar situation, a community mental health worker may be called upon to deal with a bright male youth who is socially withdrawn, extremely tense, and very talkative. In such a case, one of the possible defense mechanisms the youth might be employing to deal with underlying sexual conflicts is *intellectualization*. By shutting out emotion stimulated by early sexual concepts, he is able to deal with his sexual conflicts. Now, with an increased adolescent sex drive, his attempts to divert his drives into studying are failing. Concentration on intellectual activity has been disrupted by an increasing urge for social involvement, as previously successful defenses give way to anxiety.

The important thing to remember about defense mechanisms is that they are unconscious and operate automatically. Everyone uses them, and they become obvious and are termed "abnormal" only when they fail. Persistent failure leads to a further search for defenses and eventually may end in the development of an abnormal psychiatric behavior syndrome.

Treatment

The process of helping people to cope with their symptoms of anxiety can take a number of forms. If the anxiety is debilitating, professional intervention is usually indicated.

A number of approaches appear to have value for the treatment of anxiety. Insight-oriented approaches (e.g., psychodynamic, cognitive therapies), behavior modification, and pharmacotherapy may all prove helpful in the alleviation of anxiety conditions. The choice of therapy will depend upon the background and theoretical bias of the therapist, as well as the type of patient and severity of the symptoms presented.

Insight Therapy.   Insight therapy is a long-term effort designed not only to overcome the symptom, but, through interpretation, to expose the cause and correct it. Often the focus of such insight therapy is on helping the client become aware of the nature of his/her internal conflict, which is posited to be the root of the anxious symptomatology. Psychodynamic psychotherapy exemplifies this internal conflict model of insight therapy.

A somewhat different form of insight therapy is that found in the cognitive model. Whereas previous psychotherapy models attempted to get the client "in touch" with their feelings or internal conflicts, the cognitive-based psychotherapies argue that so-called emotional disturbances are emotional only in a very tangential way. Such cognitive therapies attempt to provide the client with a number of insights. Through a variety of exercises and therapeutic techniques, the client becomes aware that (1) emotional reactions are a function of the way an individual is thinking at any one moment; (2) dysfunctional feelings (e.g., panic attack) are a result of dysfunctional thinking (i.e., cognitive distortions); and (3) challenging and changing these dysfunctional thoughts will result in the generation of reasonable, functional emotions.

Behavior Modification.   A number of theorists posit that anxiety is a conditioned (i.e., learned) response. From this orientation the prescribed regimen of treatment is to "attack" the learned, anxious behaviors directly.

One approach that has proven effective in alleviating anxiety reactions is *systematic desensitization.* This technique requires that the client experience a pairing of the anxiety-producing stimuli (in vivo or via mental imagery) with a state of physical relaxation. The pairings are made in a hierarchical order, beginning with the least anxiety-producing situation and gradually progressing to the most anxious condition. Since anxiety and relaxation are incompatible responses, anxiety responses decrease as relaxation responses increase. The previously learned response of becoming anxious when confronted with a particular situation is *relearned* so that it elicits a relaxed or neutral reaction.

Pharmacotherapy.   The use of tranquilizers in the treatment of anxiety has been both a blessing and a curse. On the positive side, minor tranquilizers such as diazepam (Valium®), chlordiazepoxide (Librium®), oxazepam (Serax®), and meprobamate (Miltown® or Equanil®) have been quite effective in treating the symptoms of anxiety.

Barbiturates such as Seconal® or Nembutal® may also be used when excessive anxiety prevents sleep. However, because of their addicting properties their use is restricted today. Moreover, minor tranquilizers or antianxiety agents are less apt to cause such symptoms as drowsiness, skin inflammation, and a lowering of normal social defenses, or lead to suicide, as barbiturates may do.

Minor tranquilizers are effective in containing the temporary unpleasant effects of many anxiety-producing situations, permitting the person to continue to function until the situational problem is resolved. In serious cases, they act to stabilize the patient so that psychotherapy may be undertaken.

Problems arise in the use of drugs such as Valium® or Librium® when they are employed as substitutes for effective therapeutic intervention. If a physician simply provides a prescription to control the symptoms of an anxious patient without further exploration for causal factors, the results may be quite harmful.

Instead, once rapport has been established, inquiry should determine the following:

1. Whether support and prescription is sufficient at this time to get the patient through the temporary crisis; or
2. Whether the precipitating problem is actually a self-perpetuating one and referral to a mental health professional (psychologist, psychiatrist, social worker) is indicated.

Continued prescription of minor tranquilizers as antianxiety agents without the presence of adjunctive psychotherapy is contraindicated. Rather than relieving the presence of infrequent symptoms in cases of occasional minor situational disorders, or allowing a client to curtail his or her anxiety while in therapy, the problem is merely masked. Such masking of symptoms of an untreated anxiety-related problem can lead to the development of a more pronounced emotional disorder, or even to suicide.

Furthermore, the antianxiety drug user often develops a tolerance to its effect and requires a higher dosage, making possible the development of dependence and addiction. Also, accidental use in combination with alcohol may result in a serious or even fatal sedative reaction. Thus, in cases in which prescription of an antianxiety agent seems indicated for more than a brief period of time, a psychotherapeutic evaluation is warranted. This will establish whether there is a need for therapy and will also review drug use to determine whether its effect is the appropriate one in the circumstances.

Dealing with the Anxious Client

Interacting with anxious individuals is frequently a difficult task. Because they tend to be uneasy and uncomfortable, they may also become irritable or project their anger onto the interviewer. If no physical cause for their physical symptoms can be found, they may react with resentment when it is implied that their physical problems have no organic basis.

In responding to a client's hostility, the interviewer may react negatively, further worsening the communication problem. A worker who is called upon to do many intakes in a short period of time can easily forget that anxiety symptoms are real and thus become resentful of the anxiety-prone client.

To avoid this predicament, the interviewer must make an effort to comprehend the difficulties the person is experiencing when faced with anxiety-provoking situations, even when these may be vague or undefinable. If the health worker remains calm and patient with an anxious client, much can be done to alleviate the uneasiness and irritability until more extensive treatment can be initiated. Immediate help can take the form of brief supportive efforts, such as providing a relaxed atmosphere, permitting emotional release, interspersing neutral questions with pointed ones so as not to raise anxiety, and offering reassurance.

If the tense person is given the opportunity to relax, perhaps smoke while being encouraged to give a full account of his or her concerns and problems, his or her anxiety level will usually go down. When this occurs, if the worker should phrase questions with care, avoiding direct or close-ended ones in favor of indirect inquiries combined with neutral topics, such as talking about the client's job or other interests, the stage is set for *limited* reassurance.

Broad reassurance is usually worthless and may even increase anxiety. Most people are not affected by such meaningless statements as "Everything will be OK." However, more specific supportive statements can do much to alleviate anxiety.

Illustration 1

Client: "I just feel so nervous that I don't know if I can stand it for much longer without cracking up. These shakes are just driving me crazy."

Interviewer: "I can see you're at the end of your rope and that you might think your nervousness will never end. But now that you've come here I'm sure we can do something for you. It may take a little time, but now we are in a position to work with you, to start at least exploring how we can begin to curb your shakes."

Illustration 2

Ct.: "Now that the people here haven't found anything seriously wrong with me, I don't know what I'm going to do about this sudden spell of jitteriness and uneasiness."

Int.: "Well, now that the worry concerning your possible illness is off your mind, you should start feeling better in a couple of days. It's natural to be a bit upset as well as happy when nothing serious is found wrong. People generally respond in such a way. However, the time you've spent here has started to help you relax and you're beginning to look better already. Naturally, if you need some further help, you can always come back."

Summary

Anxiety is involved in many emotional disorders and is present as a symptom in forms of minor stress. It can precipitate a physical illness, be the product of one or accompany it, making the physical curative process more difficult.

Anxiety can sometimes be disguised or be so exaggerated that mis-diagnosis of the client (e.g., myocardial infarction instead of an acute anxiety reaction) results. When present, it can make dealing with a patient a real burden for hospital personnel. In mental health centers, clients with either symptoms or defense patterns that result from the presence of anxiety can be equally difficult.

If health workers can recognize some of the forms and effects of anxiety, they can be more effective in offering help. The combination of awareness and sensitivity in the worker will do much to help the client to overcome some of the crippling effects of anxiety.

6 / *depression*

Depression is a powerful enemy. An individual's primary human drives and forces may be stunted or dramatically altered by severe depression. When depressed, a person may see life in a totally negative way and may lose the sex drive, the desire to eat, and the ability to sleep, or even reach the point that suicide seems an attractive solution to personal problems.

However, depression is a universal phenomenon, and it is not confined to one age or class. Abraham Lincoln feared to carry a gun because his frequent fits of depression might have tempted him to commit suicide. Winston Churchill referred to his depressive episodes as his "black friend." Excessive grief and depression are thus often found even among the powerful and privileged.

Obviously, mood disorders are quite common; they can afflict the rich and the poor, the famous and the unknown, the child and the adult. Because they are debilitating and may even lead to suicide or homicide, it is essential to understand the basic concepts that have been developed to explain depression and its causes.

What Is Depression?

Everyone has experienced *minor* forms of depression at certain points in life. Debilitating clinical depression is less common. However, health practitioners frequently encounter clients suffering from symptoms of pathological (exaggerated) depression.

Often depressive reactions appear quite logical and comprehensible given the circumstances experienced. One such example would be reflected in the case of the forty-five-year-old woman who had recently lost both her husband and two children in a plane crash and who consequently fell into a state of depression. Under the guidelines offered in the DSM III, this individual might be diagnosed as experiencing an adjustment disorder with depressed mood. Such adjustment reactions are manifested by many who experience the loss of a job, or a lover, or the disappointment of failure or rejection.

Often, however, individuals manifesting depressive symptoms do not appear to be responding to a specific set of precipitating factors or stressors. Instead, they appear to be reacting completely out of proportion to the actual stress or loss. These examples of prolonged melancholy might more clearly represent the complex affective disorder of depression.

Characteristics of Depression

Depression is characterized by a number of symptoms. The essential feature is either a dysphoric mood, or loss of interest or pleasure in all, or almost all, of the usual activities and pastimes previously enjoyed. The symptoms most often associated with a major depressive episode are psychomotor agitation or retardation, sleep disturbance, decreased energy, feelings of worthlessness and guilt, changes in sexual interest or performance, difficulty in concentrating or thinking, thoughts of death and suicide, change in appetite and weight, and convictions of hopelessness. Since not all individuals experiencing depressive reactions exhibit each of the aforementioned symptoms, the diagnostic criteria listed in the DSM III proves helpful in identifying major depressive episodes (see table 6.1).

Mixed or Masked Depressions

Though the characteristics of depression are fairly well established, in some instances a mood disturbance may be masked by certain physical symptoms and vague complaints. One clue to masked depression might be the client's recent visit to a physician or community health center because of a variety of general, though minor, complaints (fatigue, stomach pain, constipation, headaches), or a phobia (irrational fear) about contracting cancer or heart trouble at some future time.

The potential problems that can result when depression is overlooked or underestimated by the health professional may include self-mutilation, suicide, and homicide (as when a depressed person kills himself and family).

Observation and Questioning

In some cases the signs and symptoms of depression will be quite evident. If an individual keeps repeating that all is lost, continually wrings his or her hands in agitation, and says he or she has felt poorly for weeks and does not know why, referral for further evaluation and treatment of depression is clearly indicated. However, in many instances, a pattern of symptoms, or syndrome, indicating serious depression may require special alertness on

Table 6.1. Diagnostic Criteria for Major Depressive Episode*

Diagnostic criteria for major depressive episode:

A. Dysphoric mood or loss of interest or pleasure in all or almost all usual activities and pastimes. The dysphoric mood is characterized by symptoms such as the following: depressed, sad, blue, hopeless, low, down in the dumps, irritable. The mood disturbance must be prominent and relatively persistent, but not necessarily the most dominant symptom, and does not include momentary shifts from one dysphoric mood to another dysphoric mood, e.g., anxiety to depression to anger, such as are seen in states of acute psychotic turmoil. (For children under six, dysphoric mood may have to be inferred from a persistently sad facial expression.)

B. At least four of the following symptoms have each been present nearly every day for a period of at least two weeks (in children under six, at least three of the first four).

    (1) poor appetite or significant weight loss (when not dieting) or increased appetite or significant weight gain (in children under six, consider failure to make expected weight gains)

    (2) insomnia or hypersomnia

    (3) psychomotor agitation or retardation (but not merely subjective feelings of restlessness or being slowed down) (in children under six, hypoactivity)

    (4) loss of interest or pleasure in usual activities, or decrease in sexual drive not limited to a period when delusional or hallucinating (in children under six, signs of apathy)

    (5) loss of energy; fatigue

    (6) feelings of worthlessness, self-reproach, or excessive or inappropriate guilt (either may be delusional)

    (7) complaints or evidence of diminished ability to think or concentrate, such as slowed thinking, or indecisiveness not associated with marked loosening of associations or incoherence

    (8) recurrent thoughts of death, suicidal ideation, wishes to be dead, or suicide attempt

C. Neither of the following dominate the clinical picture when an affective syndrome (i.e., criteria A and B above) is not present, that is, before it developed or after it has remitted:

    (1) preoccupation with a mood-incongruent delusion or hallucination...

    (2) bizarre behavior

D. Not superimposed on either Schizophrenia, Schizophreniform Disorder, or a Paranoid Disorder.

E. Not due to any Organic Mental Disorder or Uncomplicated Bereavement.

* From the *Diagnostic and Statistical Manual of Mental Disorders (DSM III)* by the American Psychiatric Association. Copyright 1980 by the American Psychiatric Association. Reprinted by permission.

the part of the worker. Correct diagnosis is much less difficult when observation and questioning are carefully directed toward uncovering hidden signs and symptoms. Verbal and nonverbal clues suggesting that the client has (1) a distorted sense of time (i.e., sees time as "hanging heavy," slow to pass); (2) a hopeless view of the future and personal aspiration ("what's the use?"); (3) difficulty with sleep (e.g., falling asleep, staying asleep, sleeping comfortably); and (4) limited energy and general motor retardation (e.g., sluggish, slowed down, without energy, overwhelmed by minor activities and tasks) signal the existence of a major depressive episode.

Even before attempting questions, an attentive interviewer can pick up a number of warning signs through close observation of the client's mood, rate of responding and speaking, and general consistency of behavior:

1. Does the person appear sad, low, withdrawn, or tearful?
2. Is his or her rate of speech slow?
3. Does the client seem to have difficulty considering his or her response to an issue before actually commenting on it?
4. If the client has been seen before, is he or she now more tense or withdrawn?

If some of these clues to possible depression are present, further questioning is indicated. Such follow-up interrogation would be designed to determine whether the person is experiencing only a temporary low or—to some degree—is in fact suffering from a persistent mood disorder.

The following questions are typical of those normally employed to uncover symptoms:

1. How have you been feeling lately? How long have you been feeling poorly? What is your general outlook when you get up in the morning? (Frequently when an individual suffers from depression, he or she feels low in the morning but becomes more active as the day goes on.) Do you feel better in the evening than in the morning?
2. How are you sleeping? Do you feel tired or fatigued during the day?
3. Is your interest in food diminishing? Have you lost or gained any weight recently?
4. How do you feel about yourself as a person today?
5. How do you feel about the future? Do you believe you have an impact on what the future holds for you?
6. Do you ever feel life isn't worth the effort?
7. Have you ever been so blue that you felt you must do something about it, perhaps something drastic? (If the answer to this is affirmative, additional questions should be asked. See the following section on depressive syndromes.)

In addition to the questions outlined, we have found the use of a simple checklist or inventory at the time of initial interview provides valuable data from which to assess the client's affective response level. One such measure is the Beck Depression Inventory (BDI) (Beck, 1979). This instrument has been demonstrated to be a relatively simple yet reliable mood-measuring device, which not only detects the presence of depression but provides a means of rating its severity. The measure is a simple multiple choice questionnaire that takes a few minutes to complete and can be completely self-administered and self-scored. The reader seeking a more detailed description of the scale is referred to the original presentation (Beck, 1979), or to a helpful contemporary work on depression and cognitive therapy, *Feeling Good* (Burns, 1981).

Depressive Syndromes

Since mood disturbances can be labeled and categorized in a number of ways, there is a great deal of controversy over how serious depressive syndromes should be defined. Historically, depression has been categorized dichotomously.

One approach was to distinguish psychotic and neurotic depression. Psychotic depression was defined as that in which the individual experienced severe personality disturbances marked by frequent loss of contact with reality, presence of delusions (systematized false beliefs), and hallucinations (experiencing things that are not present).

The depressive psychotic normally requires hospitalization, since the depression is often severe and generates a high potential for suicide. When auditory or visual hallucinations are present, the theme running through them may often be connected with dying, sinfulness, and punishment. The following statements by psychotic depressive individuals are typical:

> "I'm being punished because I'm the worst person in the world."
> "My body is slowly deteriorating."
> In middle and upper economic class individuals: "I'm so poor that I need to beg."
> "I'm so totally useless and worthless I feel like a parasite; I've never been of any worth."

Unlike the psychotic, the person classified as being within the neurotic depressive range rarely requires hospitalization. Neurosis is a mild personality disorder in which there is no gross disorganization or loss of contact with reality. Thus, in neurotic depression the state of sadness or hopelessness rarely becomes severe. Despite his or her depression, the neurotic functions more or less normally, responding appropriately to his or her environment while being free of the kinds of delusions that characterize the psychotic person.

Consequently, the primary distinction between neurotic and psychotic depression is that, although both disorders exhibit depression as a predominant symptom, in the latter its manifestations are more severe, and impairment of ability to understand, maintain contact, and respond to the environment is greater.

A second dichotomy compared endogenous versus exogenous depression. The former was depression which was internally generated, perhaps genetic and/or biochemical; whereas the latter was triggered by emotional conflicts and external stress.

The DSM III deviates from these historical dichotomies and lists depression as a subcategory within the class of major affective disorders. Major affective disorders include a number of subcategories (see table 6.2). The primary division is between affective disorders which include manic episodes (i.e., bipolar disorders) and those absent of such manic expression (major depression). Mania is almost a mirror image of depression. In this state, the person is frequently grandiose, oblivious to the feelings of others, verbally abusive, careless in dress, boisterous, demanding, and disoriented. (Initially, the manic individual often may appear euphoric, outgoing and quite ebullient; diagnosis of psychopathology may be difficult for the untrained person at this point).

Suicide

When persons are totally convinced that life is hopelessly unbearable and they themselves are worthless, then the only "logical" course of reaction may appear to be the termination of pain and life through suicide. Depression is not the only condition for suicide. Researchers have demonstrated that suicide can often be a result of alcoholism, addiction, psychosis, or the

Table 6.2. Diagnostic Criteria for Major Affective Disorders DSM III (1980)*

Bipolar Disorder. Essentially represents a condition in which the individual alternates between extreme moods of depression and elation. The disorder may be further categorized as of mixed, manic, or depressed forms.

mixed. Current or most recent episode involving the full symptomatic picture of both manic and major depressive episodes, intermixed and rapidly alternating every few days. Depressive symptoms are prominent and last at least a full day.

manic. Currently or most recently manifesting a manic episode.

depressed. Had had one or more manic episodes and is currently (or most recently) in a major depressive episode.

Major Depression. Demonstrates one or more major depressive episodes (see characteristics in table 6.1) and has never had a manic episode.

---

* From the *Diagnostic and Statistical Manual of Mental Disorders (DSM III)* by the American Psychiatric Association. Copyright 1980 the American Psychiatric Association. Reprinted by permission.

experience of long standing pain or terminal disease. It is unquestionably true, however, that depression and suicide are often inextricably linked. When depression goes unrecognized, untreated or is inadequately managed, the risk of self-destruction is increased.

As human service professionals, we must begin to alert ourselves to the early detection signals of suicide. People attempting suicide often provide evidence of experiencing pervasive feelings of loneliness, self-defeat, and unbearable pressure. Research has indicated that a person exhibiting signs of *haplessness* (i.e., "evidence" that *fate* has turned against them—bad luck); *helplessness* (i.e., inability to resolve the real and perceived problems facing them); and *hopelessness* (i.e., not only is life useless/valueless, but it cannot be reversed) are clearly high risk and potentially suicidal individuals.

Bringing up the issue of suicidal thoughts with the depressed client is necessary, but this must be done with care to avoid offense or to precipitate attempts at suicide that result in self-mutilation. The following are a few illustrations of how the question of suicide may be introduced:

Illustration 1: Via Biological Needs
    Client: "I just don't feel myself. I don't want to eat anything. I'm not interested in sex. ...."
    Interviewer: "The sexual drive and the basic desire to eat in order to exist are usually fairly strong and ingrained in human beings. People who don't eat and have suddenly lost interest in sex sometimes feel this way because they don't feel life is worth the effort anymore. Have you had feelings like this?"

Illustration 2: Via Social Instincts
    Ct.: "I just don't care anymore. I don't feel like doing anything. I don't want to go out anymore. I just feel like...well, lonely and yet I'm not up to being with people."
    Int.: "Your behavior seems a lot different from what it was before, Jane. Being with and enjoying other people is a very big part of life. Some people who retreat from others also feel they really don't want to put any more effort into life. They sort of feel life just isn't worth the bother anymore. Have you ever had such thoughts?"

If the person does eventually admit to suicidal thoughts or an inclination to self-mutilation, further questioning to determine the degree of danger is indicated. This can be done simply by asking such questions as:

Have your thoughts about suicide (dying, ending it all) been fleeting or do they persist?
Have you ever fantasized about how you would do it?
Do you have the means at your disposal to fulfill this fantasy?
Have you ever come close to doing it?
Have you actually attempted it?
Has anyone in your family or a friend ever attempted or committed suicide?

The more thinking and planning about suicide the person has done, the greater the danger. If suicide is not foreign to the client; that is, if a friend or relative has attempted or committed it, or the client has self-mutilated, the potential for self-injurious behavior is stronger.

Other clues to the danger of suicide that are possibly more clear and dramatic, but paradoxically are often overlooked, are a dramatic improvement in the mood of a very depressed person, accompanied by words and actions indicating a final leave-taking. If an agitated or depressed person suddenly becomes peaceful and calm, this may indicate that a decision to end it all has been made. Worry has been cast aside because the end of all troubles is in sight.

Whenever a seriously depressed person's behavior alters markedly, perhaps characterized by giving away possessions, returning borrowed items, making out a will, or remarking that his or her problems "soon will end," the danger of actual suicide increases.

Though these acts and remarks may seem clear warning signs, it is unfortunate that they are often ignored. Friends or relatives of the depressed person may attribute the signs to the desire to attract attention—to "acting," or to "being dramatic." The fallacy that a person who has injured himself or herself earlier or threatened suicide is unlikely to make another attempt is widely accepted.

Another aspect of this problem that the worker may encounter is coping with an agitated or depressed person who is about to attempt suicide or self-mutilation. This may take the form of threatening to jump from a hospital window, to inflict a wound with a pointed object, or to ingest poison.

In such instances, an impulsive move toward the suicidal person may actually precipitate the act of self-mutilation. After sending for assistance, the worker can help to keep the situation under control by taking a few simple steps.

1. Keep everyone as quiet as possible. (Noise may make the person more anxious.)
2. Attempt to make voice or eye contact with the person; speak in an even, steady voice.
3. Appeal to the person's will to live; at the very least, try to involve him or her in conversation. This helps to gain time, induce calm, and encourage a return to normalcy.

Suicide need not be the tragic outcome of depression in many cases. Skilled questioning, appropriate treatment, and careful follow-up can help the depressed person to a point where self-injury no longer seems an appealing option. However, if an individual is firmly bent on the act of suicide, little can be done. Observation and treatment will have the desired effect only when applied with skill and genuine concern at a critical time, but failure to prevent the suicide is always possible.

Treatment

Depression normally is treated by three types of therapeutic methods: psychotherapy, pharmacotherapy, and convulsive therapy. These methods will be examined below, but it should be noted that two or more methods may be employed at the same time. (A severely depressed individual may be put on antidepressive drugs while receiving supportive psychotherapy.)

Psychotherapy. Therapy has long been employed to aid the depressed person to cope with and understand the debilitating symptoms of depression. Many therapeutic modalities, with varying theoretical bases, have been used with depressed patients. One of the most frequently employed and widely researched is cognitive psychotherapy.

Though this approach reflects a particular theoretical school of thought, many of its concepts and techniques are common to other major therapeutic modalities. A major premise of this approach is that *pathological depression is a function of irrational, dysfunctional thinking and cognitions (i.e., ways of interpreting or giving meaning to one's experiences).* Specifically, cognitive therapy posits that when an individual is feeling depressed, his or her thoughts/cognitions are dominated by pervasive negativity. Further, these negative thoughts contain *gross* distortions of reality and are based upon *faulty* thinking processes. Themes such as the following are typical:

1. Self-derogatory opinions
2. Self-criticism
3. Negativism about the future
4. Harsh interpretation of current incidents
5. Negative evaluation of one's own abilities, duties, and responsibilities

In addition to such negative themes, the depressed individual often employs cognitive processes that tend to distort reality in support of his/her self-damning, negativistic view of self and the world. *Selectively attending* to negative evidence, while *discounting* positive experiences; *overgeneralizing* from one experience of failure or rejection and *catastrophizing* (i.e., taking real disappointments and mentally magnifying them to the point where they are perceived as unbearable) are but a few of the cognitive distortions exhibited by the depressed individual.

The cognitive therapist strives to provide a therapeutic climate in which the client feels accepted and supported, with the goal of assessing and correcting the unrealistic thoughts that appear to be the cause of depression. The therapist employs a series of directed, educative techniques aimed at assisting the client to take steps to recognize and prevent irrational negative thoughts. The client is guided to understand how he or she is encouraging self-defeat by exaggerating minor difficulties; by accepting broad, negative self-evaluations; and by depreciating personal assets. Emphasis may also be given to activities that will prevent the development of thoughts leading to depression and will build a positive self-image.

Pharmacotherapy. Antidepressant medication has revolutionized the treatment of depression. At a minimum, it enables the client to live with depression until supportive, cognitive, or psychoanalytic psychotherapy can have an impact.

Before pharmacotherapeutic antidepressant agents became available, management of dangerous hyperacute mania and depression was exceedingly difficult. And communication with the extremely depressed person was a severe problem.

Currently there are two main classes of drugs successfully employed in the treatment of major depressive episodes. *Tricyclic antidepressants* such as Tofranil®, Elavil®, and Sinequan® are a group of compounds that appear to alleviate depressive symptoms via the biochemical "reuptake" process. The explanation for their effectiveness is that depression often occurs when the nerve cells reabsorb serotonin (a neurotransmitter) too quickly, thus inhibiting neural conduction. The tricyclics are thought to interfere with the neurons' ability to absorb the serotonin. The remaining serotonin thus facilitates neural impulses and as such alleviates the depressive symptomatology.

The second major class of drugs employed with depression is that of the *monoamine oxidase (MAO) inhibitors* (e.g., Nardol®, Parnate®). Rather than affecting the reuptake of the neural transmitters, the MAO inhibitors function to inhibit the working of MAO, which is a substance credited with the ability to break down neural transmitters (i.e., serotonin). Thus, if MAO is inhibited, the reserve of serotonin will remain high and alleviate the depressive reaction.

While each of these drugs can prove effective in the alleviation of depressive symptoms, they do have their drawbacks. Both groups produce negative side effects such as dryness of the mouth, constipation, dizziness, and insomnia. The MAO inhibitors, however, are potentially the more dangerous of the two groups. People using MAO inhibitors must avoid certain foods (e.g., cheese, chocolate), since the substance tyramine contained in these foods can combine with the medication to create a sharp sudden elevation of the person's blood pressure, resulting in a possible stroke or death.

In addition to these negative side effects and the reality that these drugs do not prove effective with all clients, antidepressant medication fails to act quickly and that proves to be a major limitation to its usefulness. Consequently, the severity of the depression or the threat of potential self-harm or suicide may necessitate the employment of a more dramatic form of treatment.

Convulsive Therapy

Since the appearance of effective antidepressants ten years ago, convulsive therapy is used much less often. However, in cases of serious depression it may be the most effective therapeutic modality that can be employed. It is also the treatment of choice when *antidepressants have failed, or there is an imminent danger of suicide and complete supervision until drugs are effective is impossible to provide.*

There are three types of convulsive therapies, two of which involve the inhalation or injection of a drug. Drug convulsive therapy is rarely employed today. A third method, electroconvulsive therapy (ECT), is the most commonly used and best known of the convulsive therapeutic approaches.

How convulsive therapy actually effects alleviation of depression is still not fully understood. One theory holds that the depressed patient desires to die, and ECT in some way makes him or her face the reality of death, causing some improvement in his or her condition. Another explanation is connected with concepts of punishment and guilt. After receiving shock treatment the patient feels he or she has atoned for transgressions against family, God, or the like. On the other hand, organic theories center on the way ECT alters chemical neuronal activities. Another, less sophisticated theory involves the belief that many a truth is exposed in jest, as in the tongue-in-cheek statement by one psychologist that "the patient learns that he better get well or they'll continue to shock the daylights out of him."

Table 6.3. Electroconvulsive Therapy Procedure

Individual is restrained and mouth gags are inserted to prevent injury to tongue or teeth.

Muscle relaxants are injected to reduce intensity of convulsion and thus reduce incidences of bone fracture. (In some cases a barbiturate is injected intravenously immediately prior to the relaxant to alleviate the fear that individuals have resulting from the ECT procedure.)

Electrodes placed on person's temple; an alternating current of 70 to 130 volts is passed between them for a duration of .1 to .5 second.

Three treatments a week for two to three weeks is the average course of treatment.

Individual is kept under observation for the first hours after treatment since a period of posttreatment confusion usually lasts this long.

Individual is advised about some of the possible temporary side effects in order to avoid unnecessary future anxiety:
a. For females: amenorrhea for one to two months.
b. Impairment of recent memory for up to three weeks.

Administration of ECT today is a relatively safe procedure that usually takes place in the hospital (see table 6.3). There are a number of organic contraindications to ECT's use, such as TB or heart failure. For this reason, a physical and medical history is a necessary prelude to administration of ECT. Electroconvulsive therapy also has been ineffective in cases involving neurotic or schizoaffective depressions. As a method of treatment, ECT may be chosen when danger of suicide is great, quick results are sought (antidepressants sometimes take several weeks to produce a true mood alteration), or other techniques have failed. It remains a dramatic approach to be applied when very dangerous illness has resisted other forms of treatment.

Treatment of Situational Depression

The types of treatment outlined in the preceding sections are frequently supplemented by changes in the client's environment, brought about by the direct intervention of the worker. This is particularly important when there is an overwhelming situational problem in which the depression is an understandable reaction after repeated failures by the client to deal successfully with his or her problems.

Social change should not be discounted in favor of efforts at personality change. Often both assume equal importance. In some cases, helping to effect social change may even be the primary function of the worker. Too often when an individual comes to a community clinic for help, it is assumed that the sole task is to lift the depression, when this is the major symptom manifested. However, unless the worker does a careful intake evaluation, he or she may overlook an important underlying social cause that triggered the depression.

For example, if the client is depressed because she is living in an apartment where her children are threatened by peeling lead paint and rat infestation, helping her to adapt to such a situation would be inappropriate. In addition to helping her recover so she can become sufficiently assertive to deal with the landlord herself, she should also be supported by the clinic staff in seeking immediate action. Possibly the worker will help in taking action against the landlord to force repairs. While this is done, welfare may need to be contacted to temporarily relocate the family.

Obviously, community workers must see themselves not only as therapists, but also as social advocates for their clients when the occasion warrants. Unfortunately, many workers see social intervention as less important than psychotherapeutic techniques. Apart from the harmful results of such attitudes, they are elitist and tend to undermine the concept of effective total community support for the client who seeks help.

Summary

Normal depression is experienced by everyone at some time or other. It is not a product of the age, but rather an outgrowth of the human experience itself.

When it passes without debilitating intensity, the person who is subjected to it may be the better for the experience. Possibly its appearance is involved with the separation from a loved one or a lost object or dream. Whatever the reason, depression is a normal reactive experience in many situations.

However, persistent or exaggerated depression due to some physical or psychological cause is a reason for concern. Therefore, workers must be alert to the ways it commonly manifests itself, as well as sensitive to the subtle manner in which it can appear, such as vague somatic complaints.

In most cases, alertness to the signs of depression can avert danger or tragedy. However, because of the physical-illness orientation of many professionals in hospital community health settings, even the most blatant symptoms of depression may be ignored or misinterpreted. It is to be hoped that this will prove a temporary situation that will disappear as guidelines for recognizing and uncovering depression are more widely disseminated.

part three

intervention

7 / *counseling*

Helping a client with an emotional or medical problem is rarely a straight-forward task.* Even when the worker is able to make a correct diagnosis quickly and easily, the goal of assisting the client to regain physiological and functional normality can be difficult to reach.

There are many reasons why clients resist understanding and treatment of their problems. Some fear to admit to personal difficulties, while others may derive secondary gain from being incapacitated. Reasons for being resistant to help vary widely.

Whatever the reason, many people are unable to make the choices or decisions that are essential to problem-solving techniques. Negative reactions to the advice offered by workers, family, or friends are common, and must be overcome before successful treatment can be initiated.

When intervention is resisted by the client, the worker, like a friend or family member, may be tempted to turn away from the client.

"If he refuses to take my advice, there's little else I can do."

"If she's given up and doesn't really want to do anything to get out of her depression, I'm certainly not going to waste time with her!"

However, successful counseling requires that the client be permitted to set the pace, no matter how slow progress may appear to be. The counselor must display patience and understanding, while assuring the client sympathetic support and assistance.

What Is Counseling?

Varied popular fictional portrayals of the psychologist or psychiatrist have encouraged most of us to conjure up strange and almost mystical images of the process of counseling. While the expectations of each client entering the

---

* For further discussion of counseling, in addition to this chapter see appendix A, "Counseling Keystones."

counseling office may vary, they often include images of couches, bearded men, and mind reading. True, a number of counselors are men who might even employ couches (or recliners) and wear beards. However, though having mind reading prowess is obviously well beyond the capabilities of even the most competent of counselors, the myth of the counselor being an "all-knowing" person somehow persists in the minds of some.

The particulars of what constitutes counseling is to a large extent a function of the personal characteristics of the counselor and the client, the training and orientation of the counselor, and the nature of the presenting problem. However, cutting across the personal uniqueness of the counselor and client, or the varied theoretical models employed (e.g., behavioral, psychodynamic, existential), counseling is essentially an interpersonal process of a helping sort. In counseling, a professional attempts to help the client or patient develop or rediscover his or her problem-solving skills by using a variety of techniques and approaches that are initiated within the context of this helping, facilitating relationship and interpersonal exchange.

Though the content and pace of this process will vary from session to session and according to the client being treated, the counseling process cannot go forward successfully unless the following essentials are present in the client-worker relationship:

1. A workable, warm counseling relationship
2. An atmosphere of acceptance and understanding
3. A show of confidence by the counselor that the client can develop or rediscover problem-solving skills if given enough time and support

A number of authors have attempted to distinguish counseling and the counseling process from other forms of helping (e.g., spiritual direction, advice giving, and psychotherapy) by pointing to the different settings in which the various processes are employed; the severity of the problems addressed; or the intended goals of the process. We have found that the distinction made by Tyler in her book, *The Work of the Counselor*, is most appropriate for our purposes here.

The aim of therapy is generally considered to be personality *change* of some sort. Let us use *counseling* to refer to a helping process the aim of which is not to change the person but to enable him to utilize the resources he now has for coping with life. The outcome we would then expect from counseling is that the client *do* something, take some constructive action on his own behalf. Whether the need that brings him to counseling grows out of his arrival at a point in life where an important decision must be made or out of an emotional conflict that is paralyzing his ability to act, the counselor will attempt to make forward movement possible. (Tyler, 1961, p. 12)

Counseling Relationship

A common question among beginning counselors is "How do I build up a good relationship with my clients?" Phrased another way, the question is more revealing of the novice's concern: "What am I expected to *do* to demonstrate to my clients that I'm able and willing to help them?"

The neophyte counselor, like the uninitiated client, often believes the counselor must fit the image presented in the popular literature. As such, the counselor may feel that he or she *must* be the expert in all areas; or *must* appear like a mysterious, unapproachable sage; and *must* attempt to "mind read" (i.e., interpret every symbolic utterance or gesture).

It is quite common for the new counselor to feel insecure and uncertain as to what to do, or fear that his or her awkward efforts will result in failure. However, one must guard against the tendency to overcome such fear by exaggerating or "showing off" one's expertise. In soliciting the client's trust and faith in his/her skills, the counselor makes the mistake of pretending to knowledge and experience he or she does not yet possess.

When the client reacts negatively to such interpretations or appears to accept them because of dependency or fear of rejection, the relationship is off to a poor start and may even fail completely. But if premature interpretations in the counseling relationship should be avoided, what is the counselor to do to demonstrate interest and bind the relationship?

The simplest and most immediate answer to this basic question is to be authentic, respectful and supportive to the needs of the client.

Facilitative Conditions

An effective therapeutic alliance between the counselor and the person in treatment requires that the patient feel that he or she is *sincerely* accepted and *accurately* understood. As noted above such a condition demands that the counselor be authentic; respect the client; and provide for a supportive therapeutic environment.

Authentic. To be authentic implies that the counselor sheds his or her expected role or image.

Often we are tempted to feign concern or care because we believe it is the thing to do. Care and concern for the client *are* "the thing to do," but one cannot put on care or concern as one might put on a role in a play. Such therapeutic caring requires that we, as counselors, truly feel a kinship to the person before us, and exhibit the true care and concern we feel for that person in that moment. Being authentic requires that we stop hiding behind our titles or degrees or roles. Being authentic or genuine doesn't mean "spilling your guts" or "letting it all hang out." The authentic counselor is one who does not use disguises or mechanical responses to fool or manipulate his/her clients. The genuine, authentic counselor is appropriately spontaneous, nondefensive, open, and congruent in thoughts, feelings, and actions.

Respectful. In addition to being authentic and genuine, the effective counselor needs to respect the client and be able to adequately communicate this respect.

To respect another requires that we truly appreciate and value that person simply because he or she is a human being. Such an attitude is often difficult to achieve. It demands that we look beyond the behavior of a client (which we may disdain) to the basic "goodness" and "value" intrinsic to the person.

We can communicate this respect by attending to the client; demonstrating unconditional regard for them (while expressing our displeasure or appreciation for their actions); and accepting their uniqueness.

Once the attitudes and conditions of counselor authenticity and respect have been established, the counselor must then provide the supportive, facilitative environment required for therapeutic growth.

Supportive. In order for the client to grow and to identify or develop his/her problem-solving skills, the counselor must provide the client with the opportunity to talk. Such an opportunity is promoted by the counselor's use of active listening skills. As in interviewing (see chapter 1) the counselor must patiently hear what the client has to say while being alert for verbal and nonverbal clues that will later be useful in the planning and execution of successful intervention.

The counselor will often feel that mere listening to clients is tedious and ineffective, especially in the critical early stages of counseling. But even after the alliance between the counselor and the client is established, active listening remains one of the most important operations the counselor must undertake.

Rather than seeking quick and easy explanations of a client's statements or behavior, the counselor must attempt to join with the client in his or her effort to explain how he/she deals with reality and feels about the problems being explored.

As information and the client's feelings about various topics are aired, the counselor should feed back his or her observations so both parties can better understand the data. For example, the client often is not aware of deep-seated anger until it is pointed out that a particular topic causes him or her to show annoyance.

If clients are encouraged to express their opinions, describe their anxieties and fears with no concern for verbal retaliation or rejection, they will begin to see the counselor as a nonthreatening person. When this occurs, the client can proceed more quickly to assist the counselor to establish an efficient working relationship in which issues and problems can be successfully resolved.

Though the actual stages in problem-centered, short-term counseling tend to blur and overlap, they may be simply described as:

1. Initiation and exploration
2. Understanding
3. Acting

Each of the above stages involve a variety of substages or phases that are discussed below. It must be restated, however, that even though each step is presented as a discrete phase or stage, in the actual practice of counseling the stages are fluid; and counselors may find themselves moving back and forth across and within stages as dictated by the needs of the client.

Initiation and Exploration

Prior to assisting a client with the resolution of the presenting problem, the counselor must initiate the processes of relationship building and problem identification. During this phase of counseling, attention is directed to making the client feel comfortable with the relationship (i.e., *meeting*); assisting the client to disclose and problem identify (i.e., *ventilation*); and identifying resources available for problem resolution (i.e., *reconnaissance*).

Meeting. Greeting and making an initial contact with a client may seem inconsequential, but it is an important procedure. How one impresses the client on the first meeting can determine whether a productive counseling relationship will subsequently develop, or whether uneasiness and mistrust will escalate to such a degree that continuance beyond the initial session will be difficult or impossible.

In encountering the client for the first time, the counselor's greeting should be in a natural, conversational voice. This may be followed by an invitation to be seated, and the communication by the counselor of appropriate nonthreatening information.

For example, if client Foster is referred to a sex therapy clinic because of nonorganically caused impotence that induces feelings of inferiority, the mental health worker might proceed as follows at the first session.

> *Mental Health Worker:* "Mr. Foster, my name is _____. I'm a staff member here at the clinic. Won't you please sit down?" (Indicates empty chair over on side of the room.) "The referral made by Dr. _____ tells me only that you are dissatisfied with your sex life and that it is also causing you concern in the other

areas of your life. Could you tell me a bit more about the situation so I could get a better grasp on what you're experiencing?"

Jack Foster: "Where should I begin?"

M.H.W.: "Please begin anywhere you'd like."

J.F.: "I know it sounds silly, but I'm so upset and embarrassed by all of this that I just don't know where to start. I guess it's kind of silly for a grown man to act this way, isn't it?"

M.H.W.: "You do look quite upset over whatever is bothering you. It isn't at all silly for a person to be a bit confused and flustered when he comes to see a stranger about a problem that is annoying him. I wonder if you could try to tell me about the problem, though, as you did when you went to Dr. _____ about it."

J.F.: "Well, when I went to Dr. _____ I didn't go because of my sex problem, but to get a general checkup. Toward the end of the physical, I decided to ask him about it."

M.H.W.: "It?"

J.F.: "Well, the truth is I'm impotent. I guess it started in December of 1973. As I told Dr. _____ I think the problem..." (Client relates to mental health worker what he told physician earlier in the week.)

Ventilation. Once the client begins to talk, the therapeutic benefits of counseling begin to accrue. In discussing a problem with someone who is perceived as a helper, the process of expressing one's thoughts and emotions in itself provides relief. With this in mind, the counselor should give the client full reign to express his or her feelings as time permits. This is especially important in the initial stages of the first session since the patient usually appears with a rehearsed statement that is designed to explain or perhaps to justify an attitude. Once the client has begun, the worker should take care to limit questions or interruptions only to those required to facilitate the session. During this initial stage of ventilation, the use of minimal encouragement (e.g., "huh-huh," "yes," "hmm-hmm") and open questions (e.g., "Could you tell me a little more about that?") not only move the interaction along, but also open new areas for discussion and facilitate the client's self-exploration.

Reconnaissance. During the initial session or sessions, a reconnaissance or preliminary survey is made of the client's style of interaction, personal assets and liabilities, and the issues that prompted referral. Though a counselor may decide to explore particular topics during the first several sessions, in-depth discussions are not often provided at this stage. Because initial encounters must be left open to allow the newly met client to offer clues to the depth and degree of complexity of his or her problem, charging ahead on a single topic would be a mistake on the part of the worker.

Understanding

Often when one "listens" to another in the circumstance of day-to-day conversation, he/she does so with half an ear. During these conversations, we may find ourselves daydreaming, or mentally drifting away from the interaction. Further, during such interchanges, we may find that we are spending more time evaluating the person's statements or jumping to conclusions about where he/she is going with a point rather than staying actively engaged in receiving his or her information and understanding it as he or she intended.

It is important for a counselor to provide the conditions that encourage the client to open up and disclose personal information. However, for the relationship to develop, the client must feel that the counselor has been attending and is *accurately understanding* what is being disclosed. It is through the accurate reflection of this understanding back to the client, that the client begins to better understand his or her own feelings about certain things. Most people are not fully aware of how strongly or uniquely they feel about particular matters, even though they may express their opinions openly. The counselor thus seeks to increase the client's awareness of personal attitudes and why and how they affect behavior. This process is achieved through the counselor's effective use of reflection and clarification.

Reflection. One of the functions of a counselor is to assist clients to better understand their own feelings about certain things. When reflection is employed, it may be in the form of a question or by means of a simple statement that conveys the counselor's observations of a client when a sensitive area is being covered. The use of a question in response to a client's question is a reflective technique. This should not appear to be tricky, to avoid a question asked, or to put the person on the spot. Rather, it should be clearly understood only as an attempt by the counselor to elicit the client's own thoughts on the issue.

In many instances, when a question is asked in any setting, whether in school, business, or politics, the questioner already has some idea of the answer. In reflecting a question back to a client, the object is to encourage the expression of personal opinions. In addition, it functions to discourage dependence on the counselor while indicating there are various ways to deal with a problem.

Here are some illustrations of how a counselor might redirect a question to a client.

Illustration 1
> Client: "Doc, do you think I need to be hospitalized?"
> Counselor: "What do you think, Mr. _____?"
> Ct.: "I don't know. That's why I've come to you."

Coun.: "I realize you've come for help, but I wonder what your thoughts are about hospitalization?"

Ct.: "As I said, I just don't know, that's why I'm asking you."

Coun.: "Well, certainly I don't want to hold anything back from you, Mr. _____. And though I don't know you that well yet, I'd be glad to give you my impression if you still want it at the end of the session. However, even though you don't believe you have the complete answer to your own question, you've probably thought a bit about hospitalization and have some sort of feeling about it. I wonder what those feelings are?"

Illustration 2

Ct.: "Are you married?"

Coun.: "Why do you ask?"

Ct.: "No reason in particular. Just curious. Are you married?"

Coun.: "As a matter of fact, I am, but since we hadn't been talking about marriage, what do you think could have prompted the question?"

Another method of reflection involves a statement rather than a question. If tone of voice and facial expression indicate anger, it would be inappropriate to say, "How do you feel about _____?" Instead it would be more fitting to note, "You really seem quite upset about _____."

As a technique, reflection is important because it forces clients to review their own reactions. Before clients can change or modify their ways of dealing with the world, they must be led to appreciate the intensity of their own feelings, and in this process independence and self-awareness are encouraged. Before moving to point B, one should have a clear idea of where point A is; unless clients are made aware of the sources of their feelings, confusion will prevent successful modification of behavior.

Clarification. As we have seen, reflection is a technique designed to encourage clients to generate feedback on their own feelings and opinions. A second form of feedback comes from the counselor.

By listening and withholding judgment, while reflecting on the client's questions, the counselor is communicating a message by indicating that what is said will not bring rejection and that the best route to self-understanding is self-examination.

In addition to feedback resulting from the counselor's attitude and demeanor, more specific feedback is transmitted in the form of clarifications and requests that the client elaborate or expand on particular topics. At natural breaks in the session, the counselor should review what the client has said to ensure that there has been no misunderstanding or misinterpretation (see section on "transitions" in chapter 1, "Interviewing"). This will also afford the client an opportunity to see how well or how poorly he or she has been communicating.

The following statement, made when a female psychotic patient has related that she is starting to experience auditory hallucinations, is an example of clarification:

> *Counselor:* "Let me see if I understand what you've been telling me, Ms. _____. From what you say it seems that you prefer living alone rather than with your sister, and lately you've become uneasy. You've heard voices coming from outside the door of your room at the Hotel R_____ that are vague and almost inaudible, but somehow they seem accusatory to you. You indicated further that they started several months ago and are starting to make you fearful, anxious, and, as a result, you'd like to do something about them."
>
> *Client:* "That's right except I don't think I'm fearful. Just that they're getting on my nerves. If they don't stop I may do something dreadful, but I'm not afraid of whoever is doing it."
>
> *Coun.:* "In other words, it's not that you're afraid, just worried you might lose control of yourself if they bother you any longer."
>
> *Ct.:* "That's right. I wouldn't want to hurt them."

Such clarification tells the client what the counselor has absorbed and exposes possible misinterpretation, while also indicating where there may be confusion or a lack of information. When a particular area seems important and the information given is incomplete, possibly with discontinuity in the train of thought, *repression* probably is at work. In other words, the person is unconsciously forgetting details because they reflect a sensitive area (e.g., conflict surrounding high self-image). When this occurs, a gentle request for more information may be made, or if this seems inappropriate, the area may be reintroduced by the counselor later in the session.

> *Client:* (Has just related an incident in which he had an argument with his boss, but the details are sketchy.)
>
> *Counselor:* "From the way you are telling me about this incident, there's no doubt that this interaction with your boss was pretty upsetting for you. I wonder if you could tell me about it again, but this time take your time and be as detailed as possible. Sort of put me in the actual setting so I can feel that I am right in the room with you."
>
> *Ct.:* "I'd like to, but I don't know how much I can remember of it. I think I've told you all I know."
>
> *Coun.:* "Often when a person tells a story for the second time slowly, while trying to fill in even the most unimportant details, some other things that happened are recalled. There's no harm in our spending a little time on it. Why don't you begin by relating what happened to you from the moment you left for work."

Here the counselor is not only trying to get the person to remember more about the stressful event by telling it a second time, but also is requesting him to begin the story at a neutral period during the day of the argument, rather than starting in the afternoon, the actual time the dispute took place. This encourages relaxation and usually produces the desired information.

Acting

Once the client's difficulties are defined and the relationship has been established as a supportive, caring exchange, the process can enter the acting stage. In this stage the counselor's attention is drawn to the identification of a number of alternatives or solutions (i.e., problem solving); supporting the client's attempts at problem resolution (i.e., call to action); and, finally, moving the relationship toward increased client independence and eventual termination (i.e., review and termination).

Problem Solving. Assuming that the helper has "actively" listened to the client and has accurately noted the client's concerns and potential resources, the identification of strategies for resolving the problem can take place.

Often, the needed course of action appears quite obvious to the astute counselor. However, since the counseling process is more than mere advice giving, the counselor should resist simply supplying "all of the answers." If the client was one who could accept advice from others—clergy, physician, family—in his own environment, he/she would most likely not need counseling. Further, the goals of counseling, as presented here, are broader than simply resolving the presenting complaint. As noted in the introduction, the current revolution in the human services arena is one that emphasizes prevention along with remediation. Therefore, the counselor should be attempting to increase the client's problem-solving skills and sense of independence so that he/she is better prepared to avoid or resolve problems in the future (i.e., preventive focus of counseling).

To be effective, the counselor must avoid putting the client in a dependent position; rather, he or she must work with the person to discover ways of handling the problem, refraining from giving advice except when basic information is required. Even in these instances, information is given only when the counselor perceives that time will not permit waiting for the client to search for the information, or when the information needed is of a technical nature.

Call to Action. Following the identification of potential problem-solving strategies, the client must be encouraged to test out these approaches. During this stage of counseling, the counselor needs to be extremely *supportive* of the client's *efforts* and not just of his or her achievements.

Often, the unexperienced counselor may view this period in the counseling process as the "do or die" phase, that is, a phase in which his/her own competence as a counselor is put to the test. Such an attitude often results in the counselor taking the client's failures as personal failures or, worse, as attacks on his/her own professionalism.

Rarely does the client's initial efforts prove 100% successful. The counselor needs to be prepared for disappointments and setbacks, and in turn must prepare the client to expect the same. It is helpful if during this initial period of testing solutions, the counselor not only provide the client with support for his/her efforts, but help the client to view his/her experiences (successes and failures) as important information-gathering tools. From this perspective no experience is truly a failure, only a mechanism for gathering essential data for the adjustment of one's strategy. It is also helpful for the counselor to assist the client in setting clear, concrete goals that are presented in a small, graded fashion. Such a graded approach will increase the probability of success at each level of action.

Review and Termination. A brief counseling relationship usually does not result in the formation of a lasting bond between counselor and client. Despite this, the manner in which the relationship is terminated is an important and delicate process. Clients should not be abruptly or matter-of-factly terminated, as this may cause them to feel that their problem is of no real importance to the counselor.

In the final session, or toward the end of a session in instances in which the counselor has had few contacts with the client, a review of the problem and the progress made is appropriate. Such a review not only puts past counseling work in perspective and reinforces the advances made by the client, but also serves to highlight the process followed and the procedures employed. This highlighting of the process and procedures involved in the identification and resolution of the problem serves an educational function and thus supports the preventive focus of the counseling. The hope is that the client will be able to generalize from this one experience in order to use these processes and procedures in other, similar problem circumstances.

When the review is completed, a mutual decision may be made concerning further treatment. When further treatment is not required, it may be suggested that counseling is available for any future need and remaining questions, if any, discussed before bidding the client goodbye.

Case Illustration

As noted above, counseling is more than simply providing advice. Clients with specific serious problems often seek more than just keys to solutions to their problems. The following example, which includes information giving and parallels the steps of problem-solving counseling, reviews the steps discussed and is an effective method of helping people who are upset or disturbed by a critical situation.

Presenting Problem. In the illustration, the parents are seeking help because they want to know how best to deal with their child who is suffering from a fatal disease. The nature of the problem and parental concern is such that, while advice or information may be of some assistance, it will fall short of providing the parents the relief they seek. The supportive caring environment created by the counselor will allow the parents to express their feelings of anger, and their sense of frustration and general helplessness. Further, the active involvement in the problem-solving process will provide them with a mechanism for "doing" and will ultimately prove necessary for the parents' own well-being.

Greeting. Counselor introduces himself/herself to the parents, says he/she knows that their child is dying and that he/she understands that it is a very difficult time for the clients. Then he/she asks for more details about the situation.

Ventilation and Reconnaissance. Parents express their sadness, frustrations, and fears about dealing with their dying child. Also, they retrace the steps taken thus far. At this point the clients begin to feel better for two reasons: (1) they start to feel that they are being understood because they have been encouraged to describe the circumstances in their own words; and (2) they feel better by virtue of having the opportunity to express their feelings.

Reflection, Clarification, and Elaboration. The counselor deals with initial questions by centering on the clients' feelings of frustration and failure, in order to encourage further ventilation of negative feelings. He/She then repeats, at several points in the session, what the parents have related about their feelings in dealing with this stressful situation. He/She also requests elaboration of the ways in which they have already attempted to deal with the problems and the reactions they have elicited from the child. Special attention may be given at this point to the parent who has had little to say.

Problem Solving and Support for Action. Since the situation is a new and painful experience for the parents, the counselor should offer some information on what has been learned about dealing with the child who is dying. The following section from McBrearty's paper "The Child and Death" is appropriate:

> To the dying child, his illness will cause physical limitations. He no longer has the mobility he once had either due to medical restrictions or because he no longer has the physical strength. He must give up his new sense of autonomy. This may cause the child to become angry, depressed, and confused. Illness and/or treatment may be perceived as punishment. The child may have fears of retaliation for his negative behavior and feelings, and this may be

expressed in his fear of being abandoned and mutilated. The parents can help allay some of these fears by being present as much as possible. When they cannot be present, the child should be left with familiar comfort object, e.g., a favorite blanket or soft toy. Parents should encourage the child to be as independent as possible for as long as possible. This may be very difficult for the parents to do due to their own fears for the child's well-being. It is of very little sense or comfort to tell a young child that he will go to heaven when he dies. Children are not interested in this idea because they do not want to leave home or their parents. (McBrearty, 1975, p. 59).

When this information has been presented with due care for the parents' feelings, the problems and questions it raises may be approached.

1. How do parents help the child deal with his anger, depression, and confusion?
2. What can parents do to allay fears the child may have of retaliation for his negative behavior?
3. What items can parents leave with the child when they cannot be physically present?
4. How can parents avoid unnecessarily putting the child in a dependent position?
5. What can parents do to deal with their own fears, guilt, and concerns about death?

Review and Termination. During this stage, the parents are given an opportunity to review after each session the steps they have followed. In terminating, it is important to emphasize the positive manner in which the parents proceeded, and also to encourage them to accept their grief as a normal, rather than an unhealthy, reaction. Such platitudes as "Well, it is now time for you to look to the future!" have no place in the counseling setting and are to be avoided. Such generalizations and banalities are often indicative of the counselor's own anxiety in the situation. They may also reflect an attitude of omnipotence in the counselor's hope for a miraculous intercession while fantasizing about his/her own role as problem solver.

Only through building a good relationship with the client can questions be answered and problems solved. There are no short cuts or magic cures.

Summary

Effective counseling, like other intervention procedures we have discussed, requires skill and experience. Moreover, since allied health and human services professionals often function informally as counselors and interviewers, the established guidelines for office counseling may have to be modified in practical ways when dealing with certain client groups.

Though counseling is difficult to utilize in many health settings, the techniques covered in this chapter will serve as guides to the more common types of interpersonal encounters with clients.

We have seen that counseling is more than just being friendly, even though a warm relationship with the client is essential. Counseling, however difficult in particular cases, is a demanding process that can make working in any area of the health field more productive and meaningful.

8 / crisis intervention

The previous chapters presented a brief overview to the typical diagnostic and intervention procedures used within human services. Lengthy diagnostic procedures and long-term treatment are frequently neither necessary nor possible, though. For instance, they are often inappropriate when working with individuals who are experiencing maturational and situational crises.

Individuals experiencing crisis situations find themselves in states of emergency and as such cannot afford the luxury of long-term diagnostic or intervention procedures. These individuals need quick, short-term interventions. In addition to these situations, there are many individuals who, while needing the services of a mental health professional, simply cannot afford the services of a private therapist or resist protracted treatment in a clinic for fear of being labeled "mentally ill." For each of these situations, crisis intervention procedures appear to be the intervention modality of choice.

Crisis intervention is especially designed to provide care with minimum cost or delay. Usually this means the client will be treated by a staff member the same day attention is sought. In response to this need for emergency service, the Community Mental Health Service Act of 1963 legislated that service would be available twenty-four hours a day with a community mental health center. Further, this act required that each center, in addition to offering crises intervention and suicide prevention services, offers twenty-four hour a day walk-in service; telephone hot lines; home emergency visitation facilities; and consultation and referral services. However, even with the support of this legislation, such quick response to the need for treatment is not found in all settings.

Since crisis intervention offers a needed alternative to traditional treatment modalities, it is widely accepted today. However, crisis intervention is not a recent innovation. Though its current modified form is in some sense "new," it has precedents dating back to the 1930s.

Historical Precedents

In the broadest sense, the origins of crisis intervention date from man's earliest days. The first time one person came to another with a problem and was met with some degree of understanding, support, and active assistance, rather than being attacked for being weak, crisis intervention was born. The historical roots of the movement as we know it today can be traced to Querido's work in the 1930s; treatment concepts developed for transitional situational disorders in World War II and the Korean War (Menninger, 1948; Glass, 1954); and to the work of Lindemann (1944) in the mid-1940s.

Querido (1968) established a "psychiatric first aid service" in Amsterdam in the early 1930s. This service performed not only the more traditional function of screening admissions for the area mental hospital, but also provided support to police, physicians, and social welfare agencies. Its operations included home visits and active environmental intervention in the form of helping clients to fill their housing, financial, and employment needs.

In World War II and the Korean War, a similar first aid approach was commonly employed with military personnel suffering from "combat fatigue." This condition develops when an individual demonstrates temporary personality decompensation (a "mini–nervous breakdown") resulting from the trauma of combat. When treated traditionally, a lengthy diagnostic process and removal from military duty for treatment were the routine procedures employed. The client sometimes responded with nearly *immediate* improvement upon removal from active duty, but permanent adjustment remained in doubt, possibly because of guilt over leaving combat or other active duty.

Because of these results and the fact that time and staffing were limited, a crisis-oriented approach was developed. This philosophy emphasized assistance as close to the combat area or military unit as possible and treatment of symptoms with basic supportive techniques. Together with sedation, warm food, and interpersonal support, clients were permitted time to regain personal equilibrium to enable them to return to duty promptly.

Lindemann studied normal grief reaction. He is known particularly for his work with the survivors of the tragic Coconut Grove fire in 1943, which resulted in many deaths. One of his findings suggested that failure to express feelings of bereavement after a serious loss could lead to the development of other and more extreme personality disturbances. From this study it was evident that particular crises result in specific types of postcrisis behavior. When such behavior is understood and allowed to run its course while support is given, other patterns of behavior can be developed. This can perhaps be most clearly seen in the case of grief reaction to personal loss and adapting to the condition of loss.

Characteristics of Intervention

Caplan, a pioneer in community psychology, defines a "crisis" as "a short period of psychological disequilibrium in a person who confronts a hazardous circumstance that for him constitutes an important problem which he can for the time being neither escape nor solve with his customary problem-solving resources" (Caplan, 1964).

Zusman's definition is more detailed, but does not differ in essentials from Caplan's:

> Crisis intervention is one term that can be used to describe a whole series of recently introduced, brief treatment techniques employing a wide variety of personnel, service, organizations, auspices, and formal labels. Crisis intervention includes, for example, suicide prevention services using telephone and inperson interviews, teen-age counseling as offered through "hot-line" and "drop-in centers," pastoral counseling, brief psychotherapy offered in emergency "walk-in clinics," family dispute intervention provided by specially trained policemen, window-to-window programs, and a host of similar programs (Zusman, 1975, p. 2335).

Generally, all types of crisis intervention programs display characteristics that set them apart from the more traditional therapeutic programs.

1. Specific, current, observable difficulties are the target of the therapist. If diagnostic procedures support recommendations for longer term treatment, referral to another facility or setting will be made. However, the goal of crisis intervention is to return clients to their environment as quickly as possible with a better understanding of how to employ their personal coping mechanisms. In this way the incapacitating effect of immediate situational problems can be moderated or overcome.
2. Treatment is offered only on a *short-term* basis. This is not merely because crisis units are not designed to provide unlimited psychotherapy, but is rather a question of goals. Crisis intervention aims to provide immediate relief to the client and positive feedback to the client's environment, including his or her family. Proving to all concerned, including the client, that results are possible without such extreme life alterations as long-term hospitalization or job and education termination is the primary objective of crisis intervention.
3. Intervention may often require the services of several workers. The client is usually seen by different members of the team and may have additional interpersonal community contacts with others involved in the treatment. Since the crisis is the point of focus, the client is not encouraged to develop a binding relationship with a particular psychotherapist to the exclusion of others in the team or community setting.

Thus, relevant individuals in the client's life such as family, friends, clergy, or employer, may be asked to assist in treatment by providing information or by active involvement.

4. The staff of the crisis unit is *broad-based* and less stratified than staff in other settings. Psychologists, social workers, and psychiatrists have traditionally been responsible for conducting intake interviews and providing intervention. In crisis units, the community mental health philosophy is applied; therefore, nurses, physician's assistants, mental health workers, assistant social workers, community representatives, and other human services personnel in medical and nonmedical specialties are employed.

5. *Multimodal* approaches are used to assist the client, requiring or encouraging input from each staff member. Medical personnel may be consulted concerning the appropriateness of drug therapy; community workers may express opinions as to the social, ethnic, racial, or economic issues relevant to treatment; and group process experts may be asked to provide direct or supervisory support for work with dyads, families, or more extensively structured groups from the client's community.

6. The crisis intervention section is staffed in such a way as to permit treatment to extend over a short time, usually less than a day. Most programs are staffed twenty-four hours a day to allow clients to come at any time. This is particularly important for drug users and "late-night people" who are unwilling or unable to appear during the day.

Intervention Methodology

As we have indicated, this type of treatment is based on brief, direct intervention and support. Though the actual form of treatment will vary with different individuals and their problems, there are three main phases in most cases: assessment, planning and intervention, and termination.

Assessment. According to the Joint Information Service of the American Psychiatric Association and National Institute of Mental Health (1966), each emergency program should treat every contact as a psychiatric emergency until assessment and evaluation reveals otherwise. While the assessment procedure employed under such emergency conditions is normally shorter than that typical of a full psychiatric assessment, it is still as important. Since the potential exists for an individual in crisis to engage in self-mutilation or homicide, and/or become seriously disorganized, it is essential that all haste be given to the accurate assessment of the "here and now" condition of the client. Therefore, even though the assessment will attempt to elicit extensive background material and disposing factors, much like the psychiatric assessment, it will do so only after first identifying current issues, potential dangers, and precipitating factors.

The data acquired during this initial assessment will not only provide a basis for the planning and intervention procedures to follow, but will serve as a critical foundation for those times when hospitalization or referral are required.

It is clear that crisis intervention places special demands on the human service worker. The demand for speed and accuracy of the assessment requires that the worker keep his/her composure and be able to focus specifically on those areas that most clearly define the nature of the problem and the unique resources of the client. Often the task demands that the worker be able to identify in clear, concrete terms the form of situational or maturational crisis experienced. This necessitates that the worker not only ascertain what is actually happening (or happened) to the individual (e.g., loss of job, rape, divorce) with all of the real and specific consequences of that event, but also begin to identify the meaning or consequences perceived by the client. Table 8.1 provides an example of the intake form employed and the data collected under such a crisis situation. The data reflects the crisis experienced by a 49-year-old woman who was abandoned by her husband of 28 years.

Situational and Maturational Crises.   The assessment process will help to identify the nature of the situational or maturational crisis at hand. A situational crisis results primarily from temporary external stress that exerts pressure on the client's existing coping devices (e.g., rape, separation, pregnancy). A maturational crisis is directly related to a period of personal development and the tasks associated with that period (e.g., self-concept and peer acceptance during adolescence).

This division of crisis conditions in terms of situation or development stage is somewhat arbitrary. Often, the conditions overlap or present them-

Table 8.1. Problem Identification Worksheet

Situation	Impact	
	(Real)	(Perceived)
"Husband left me after twenty-eight years for a younger woman."	"I have to pay bills." "I don't drive." "The mortgage is unpaid." "I'm alone nights." "I don't have a car." "I am without a sex partner." "I don't know how/where to meet people."	"I will never be happy." "I must be horrible." "I must be unlovable." "People will laugh at me." "No one will love me."

selves in tandem, as might be the case with the young adult who is confronted with a vocational/career decision (maturational condition) that in turn creates marital strife and eventual divorce (situational crisis).

The following is a brief listing of potential maturational/situational crises that typically demand emergency treatment:

Acute psychotic reaction	Menopause
Criminal charges	Peer group alienation
Disability	Physical illness
Disaster	Postpartum psychosis
Divorce	Rape
Drug-induced psychosis	Retirement
Homosexual panic	Serious grief reaction
Impotency	to loss
Lawsuit	School failure
Loss of status	Unemployment

Implied throughout this discussion of assessment is the need for the crisis worker to be able to identify the *real* versus the *perceived* problem experienced by the client. While such delineation is always important in providing clinical intervention, it is essential in the case of crisis intervention. Individuals in crisis often elevate their real, concrete problems to the point of experiencing the *unbearable, intolerable crisis*. Individuals in crisis often exhibit a distorted, unrealistic view of the real meaning or impact of the situation in which they find themselves. Although being confronted with *real* problems that require adaptation and personal cost in the process of problem solution, the individual in crisis fails to see the situation as simply problematic or inconvenient.

As previously noted in table 8.1, the fact that a married woman loses her husband does, in fact, demand extensive adaptation on the part of the woman. Losing one's husband creates a number of real problems and inconveniences (e.g., how to support one's self, pay the mortgage, get transportation). While these real problems are not to be treated lightly or dismissed by the individual or the crisis worker, they are resolvable and thus need not be catastrophized. The crisis, therefore, is more apt to be generated, not by these real, difficult, yet resolvable problems, but by the individual's faulty beliefs or perceptions about the problems (e.g., "This is so horrible I can't survive!" or "What's the use of living—without Ted, I just can't be happy!").

It is essential for the crisis intervention worker to help the client distinguish the real from the perceived problems and begin to outline problem resolution strategies for each of the *real* concerns so identified.

Planning and Intervention. Once assessment is made and referral is determined to be unnecessary, plans may be made for practical and direct intervention. The actual intervention will vary according to the skills, training, and creativity of the helper and the specific nature of the presenting problem. In general, however, such intervention will focus on the recent precipitating event and the resultant problem. Such a focus will thus avoid the time- and energy-consuming process of attempting to identify possible underlying causes for the crisis.

The strategy normally includes suggestions and active, direct assistance by the crisis intervention worker in developing a plan to utilize personal assets and environmental supports, as well as mustering new or untapped resources. We have found that the use of a force field analysis technique, such as that presented in table 8.2, often proves quite helpful at this stage of intervention.

Because of the essential emergency nature of the situation, the worker cannot afford to rely totally on nondirective, reflective methods. This is not to suggest that the worker exclude the client in the process of planning, but rather that the worker take the primary responsibility for helping to resolve the immediate crisis situation. Throughout the planning and intervention processes, it is essential that the client be provided with honest information and a clear idea of the plan of action to be followed. Providing such information and guidelines will help to focus the client on the fact that something is being done and thus help to reduce personally experienced states of panic. Further, during the initial planning and early efforts at intervention, the worker should attempt to establish the availability of family supports and contact relatives and/or friends where appropriate.

Crisis intervention personnel are not normally concerned with any unconscious defense mechanisms the person may be using, or unobservable intrapsychic disequilibrium that underlies the personality problem. The attention of the worker is restricted to the client's observable coping mechanisms and the community's available resources. Thus, an attempt is made at identifying the typical way an individual confronts a problem and which community resources are used (e.g., when anxious, the client may find it helpful to talk extensively on the phone with a friend). Such identification of typical strategies may provide the core of the therapeutic suggestions or intervention plans to follow.

While the goal is certainly reducing the immediate stress and assisting the individual through this crisis, as with all of the intervention strategies discussed, resolution is only half of the intervention plan. In addition to this remedial focus, the worker should provide a mechanism by which the client's coping skills are increased to the point at which future crisis may be averted (i.e., the preventive focus). This focus on prevention as well as remediation demands that the worker involve the client at each stage of the intervention plan and encourage the client's independent resolution of the problem presented. In addition to employing the client as an active contributor to the intervention plan, the worker should also assist the client in

Table 8.2. Procedure for Force Field Analyses

Directions

Step 1: Specify the goal or objective to be achieved. Attempt to identify the goal in clear, concrete, specific terms.
a. (example) Get a job.
b.
c.
etc.

Step 2: Identify and list all of the personal and social/environmental factors that are pushing (or assisting) you toward your goal.
positive forces
a. (example) good skills as a typist
b. (example) availability of a baby sitter
c.
d.
e.
etc.

Step 3: Identify and list those personal and social/environmental factors that are holding you back from reaching your goal.
negative forces
a. (example) poor interview skills
b. (example) no transportation/car
c.
d.
e.
etc.

Step 4: List steps that can be taken to increase the positive forces and/or reduce the negative forces.
a. (example) Take driving lessons and purchase car.
b. (example) Rehearse for interviews and practice with friends.
c. (example) Set aside time each night to continue to sharpen my typing skills.
d. etc.

---

developing a realistic plan for the future. Such a plan should address techniques for early crisis identification, reduction of precipitating stressful factors, and strengthening of successful coping skills.

Termination. When several sessions with the client have resulted in observable progress, a termination session follows. At this time the therapist reviews the crisis and how the client has dealt with it. The therapist aims to clarify the limits of the difficulty once again and to reinforce the positive steps the client has taken. Alternative ways to avoid such difficulties in the future may also be discussed. Referral to a longer-term treatment facility, such as a day hospital, or referral for therapy may be appropriate if it is apparent that the client has become increasingly disoriented even though the temporary crisis has passed.

Legal Considerations. By definition the client seeking emergency care is in crisis. A client in a crisis may attempt to employ extreme and potentially harmful, even fatal (e.g., suicide) solutions to his/her perceived crisis. Because of the possible social and legal ramifications of the behavior of such a client and the responsibility the human service worker has to both the client and society, special care must be given when treating a crisis client.

Workers who find themselves providing emergency care to a potentially suicidal individual should be sure to:

1. keep accurate and detailed accounts of dates and times of contact; procedures employed; and client reactions;
2. use procedures that are accepted as appropriate for working with such clients and that appear to be what another of equal training and experience would do;
3. document consultation with other professionals and clear evaluation of the need (or lack of need) for hospitalization;
4. generally be guided by the principle of "what is good for the client and society is what is needed."

Inpatient Crisis Intervention Units

Problems, such as drug-induced psychosis and stress reactions to adolescence, as well as others listed above, may be dealt with in an inpatient or in a short-term outpatient crisis unit. While it may seem desirable to keep the client in the community, the crisis inpatient unit has several advantages. It can handle more dangerous problems and monitor behavior more closely than an outpatient crisis unit can. For persons who manifest signs of suicidal or homicidal behavior, or who resist taking prescribed drugs, inpatient treatment may be necessary.

For example, if a youth complains of depression and has thoughts about suicide, treatment in an inpatient unit may be the best choice for successful intervention. Similarly, in the case of a middle-aged male client who says he cannot control his temper, has a history of violent outbursts, and sees a member of his own family as the cause of his difficulties, care should be taken to assess clearly how dangerous this person may be before outpatient care is attempted.

Medication is also an issue in determinating whether a client requires hospitalization. For example, if a female client who lives alone is diagnosed as an acutely depressed psychotic, it cannot be assumed that she will take her medication as prescribed. In this instance the client may see medication as useless, or may attempt an overdose, possibly in combination with another drug such as alcohol. If the client is on a high dose and is notably uncooperative about coming to the clinic or being seen at home, side effects such as drowsiness, dry mouth, pseudo-parkinsonism may develop, causing depression to deepen and putting the individual in medical danger. Agranulocytosis, another serious side effect of drugs, may appear as a mild fever but result in great harm if left undiagnosed and uncorrected.

Crisis Intervention: An Illustration

A female college sophomore who had experienced bouts of depression immediately following failure of two key examinations in her premed major was a self-referral. During her most recent crisis, she impulsively resorted to self-mutilation in the form of superficial cuts on the wrist. Her fright caused her to come to the unit for help.

Following an initial evaluation, the interviewer determined that the suicidal potential was serious but not imminent, and that quick intervention rather than immediate hospitalization was warranted.

Analysis of the problem, as outlined below, revealed areas in which active assistance could help to alleviate stress and depression.

Failed two examinations
↓
Became anxious and depressed
↓
Pondered feelings of worthlessness and uncertainty about future vocational choice without sharing these feelings with family or friends

↓

Parents expressed disappointment in her grades in a letter
↓
Decided not to go home for spring recess
↓
Continued withdrawal and depression leads to further poor academic performance
↓
Hopelessness and helplessness are experienced
↓   ↓
             Crisis

Self-injurious behavior

In the planning stage, the client and staff members worked together to develop steps designed to help improve study habits, explore alternative academic goals, and determine who in the environment could be of help during periods of extreme stress. A tutor was obtained to assist the client with her course work. The possibility of entering another less academically rigorous field than medicine was also considered. Arrangements were also made for the client to return home to discuss her feelings with her family, friends, and a clergyman to whom she related well before attending college. A meeting was held with the client's roommate and a campus counselor to see if a future crisis situation could be handled without the necessity of having the client leave school. This resulted in the client being given the option to enter group or individual counseling at a local community mental health center.

A final session reviewed the steps planned and taken, with special attention to the steady progress made; this had the beneficial effect of reinforcing therapeutic measures and of renewing the client's sense of mastery and self-confidence.

Summary

Crisis intervention is one of the more dynamic aspects of the modern community mental health movement. While it is not a complete solution for the acute emotionally disturbed client in all instances, it has often proved to be the best choice for successful treatment of certain types of clients. Such individuals might not otherwise have sought treatment, perhaps because they perceived the normal channels of a community or residential mental health program as being too slow or unappealing. Thus, crisis intervention, with its emphasis on multifaceted, brief, immediate, interdisciplinary, symptom-oriented treatment, fills a vital need today. Continuance of existing units and their expansion will greatly reduce the number of psychiatric casualties.

For a more comprehensive study of crisis intervention and the variety of problem-solving techniques used in it, see suggested readings in the bibliography.

part four

collaboration with other professionals

9 / *working with groups*

A common task for the human service professional is working together with staff, community, or client groups. Case conferences in which a number of professionals share and collaborate on the diagnosis and treatment plan for an individual require the adequate functioning of a facilitative group. Furthermore, team sessions and planning groups employ group structures and processes in order to facilitate their work. Groups are often found effective in the supervision and training of junior staff members and can even be employed as part of the treatment regimen for the client. Often, there is a need for a group when clients reach a point in their treatment where a structured interpersonal encounter with others who are experiencing similar emotional or physical problems becomes desirable.

Not only are groups a fact of life for human service professionals, they are, or can be, a very desirable and effective tool to be used in the performance of their duties. A group may be set up to assess the support a client can be expected to get from his or her environment. It can be helpful to gather the client's family and friends for a problem-solving session to determine the best way to develop the outside support a client needs to permit him or her to function outside the hospital or clinic setting. Groups can increase the worker's effectiveness and creativity in such problem solving and thus lend support to the arsenal of helping tools available to the human service professional.

Each of the aforementioned potential benefits of group functioning is predicated upon the fact that the group is operating as a facilitative, productive, and effective group. These characteristics are not simply a matter of blind luck, but rather are the result of the skills and knowledge of those actively involved. Thus, some familiarity with the basics of working effectively with groups is essential for the worker.

However, the level of skill required for physician's assistants, assistant caseworkers, and other health personnel is far short of that required for group psychotherapists, or for successful leaders of sensitivity or "T" groups, which demand a high level of training and expertise in group dynamics. Poorly or inadequately trained personnel who attempt without proper supervision to lead sensitivity groups can cause serious problems; casualties from such groups are being seen more and more often by therapists in private practice and in clinics.

Here we will cover only those factors in group process and structure that are essential to short-term experiences in working with small clusters of people. These fundamentals will also serve to outline the kinds of issues normally covered in more detail in advanced group work training. However, workers should be encouraged to seek further training in group dynamics, since it is likely that they will be more and more involved in working with groups, and to a lesser extent in providing service to individuals.

Advantages of a Group

Manpower economy is probably the most widely accepted reason for working with groups. Because of staffing shortages in the health professions, this advantage is quite appealing to most administrators and directors. However, while this is a significant advantage, it is only one of the numerous benefits of group work and should not be permitted to overshadow the unique, positive attributes of group work. It is important to emphasize this point, since working with groups has erroneously been seen by some as second-rate treatment. Individual counseling and other forms of one-to-one interventions have been considered superior only because the client receives exclusive attention in a nongroup session. Because they are different types of treatment, each with its own advantages and disadvantages, it is simplistic and misleading to see them in this manner.

What follows is just a *partial* list of overlapping advantages of group participation.

1. Participants can see how others with difficulties like their own successfully cope or struggle to handle them. The many kinds of problem-solving behaviors, including alternatives never before considered, become possible because others are trying them. Both supervisor and client are encouraged to deal with their own frustrations, conflicts, or inadequacies through the experience of observing others' struggles to overcome problems.
2. If a problem is believed to be unique, it can be overwhelming, and the possibility of improvement may be difficult to accept. However, when workers and clients see that fellow group members have similar problems, they derive therapeutic support from the realization that they are not alone.

3. Participants can feel independent as well as dependent within groups. By modeling themselves on the styles of the leader or other group members, even the newest or most diffident member can provide input for other members. This process is important because it helps to establish a basis for a transition from a position of dependence to one of independence, whether as a functioning member of the community or as a graduate allied health professional who will shortly assume the position of supervisor.
4. A participant in a group is free to experiment with new behaviors without the fear of retaliation that may be experienced outside the supportive confines of the group session. If feedback from the group shows the behavior to be appropriate, it may be generalized to the outside community or specific job setting.

Each of the assumed advantages of groups is dependent upon a number of specific factors. According to Steiner (1972), the actual productivity of a group is affected by three main ingredients, as illustrated in the following proposed formula.

Actual Productivity = (Group's Potential for Productivity) + (Positive Effects of Group Process) − (Detrimental Effects of Negative Group Process)

The potential of the group is the degree to which the group's resources (i.e., the individual members' talents, resources, abilities, characteristics) meet the demands of the task under consideration. This potential can be augmented by the somewhat unexplained synergistic effect of group process.

Positive group process not only increases an individual's energy, but also appears to stimulate group members to perform at levels of accuracy and creativity higher than might be expected given their individual talents.

Finally, the actual productivity of any one group, which up to this point has been a function of the additive effect of *Potential + Positive Group Process*, is now reduced by the *Detrimented Effects of Negative Group Process*. Negative group process often results in depletion of group and individual energy and a blocking of maximum utilization of group resources. This negative process is often the result of poor communication, contrary members, and/or inadequate leadership.

Facilitating Group Process

The goal of the human service worker functioning in a group should be to increase and maximize the benefits accrued from positive group process while at the same time reducing the detrimental impact of negative group process. Even with such intentions in mind it is clear that not every group can succeed, no matter how adept the human service worker. An error in selection, a situational crisis experienced by one or more members early in the life of a group, or any number of unforeseeable events can have a negative impact on the life and quality of a small group. However, while the presence of a skilled leader does not *guarantee* a productive group, his or her absence almost ensures failure.

Obviously, getting people to sit in a circle is merely a beginning. One must be alert to the latent content of what is said and be aware when a member is fighting the group. The role played by each member, his/her position in the group, and the overt or hidden agendas present—all need to be identified and coordinated if the group is to operate effectively.

One way of characterizing the position of group members is to place them along a dimension of "ownership." Needless to say the more one owns the group and its tasks, the more facilitative his/her involvement. Members in a group often take any one of five possible postures. The *Underminer* resents being in the group, and is actively involved in destroying the group and its processes. The *Observer*, while not actively attempting to destroy the group, does so in a slow, passive fashion. The observer is simply that, an onlooker. He/she occupies space, demands attention and consideration, but fails to contribute to the group's pool of energy and thus slowly but surely saps the group of its vital self-supporting resources. The *Responder* is an individual who is shy and restrained. The responder will be more than happy to respond when confronted or addressed—but demands that the group initiate the contact. Again, such a member often requires more group energy expenditure than is returned and thus can prove quite costly to the group's vitality and functioning. The fourth position often observed in a group is that of *Initiator*. The initiator comes to the group with a clear set of goals, aspirations, and agendas, and actively pursues these goals, seeking the support and resources of the group. The *Facilitator* is the last role or position in a group. The facilitator is one who can appreciate the value of each of the previous three roles (excluding the Underminer). The facilitator will observe and process when passive data collection is what is needed. The facilitator will respond to the specific needs of others in the group and not feel like he/she must be in control at all times or on center stage. Finally, the facilitator will have his/her own clearly identified set of agendas or goals that he/she would like addressed by the group, and be willing and able to express these goals openly to the group. Needless to say, the facilitator is just that, an individual who is capable of "reading" the various group members' positions and postures and adapt accordingly in order to maximize the positive interaction between each member of the group. The facilitator is clearly an excellent group leader.

Tasks of the Group Leader

While it is clear that a group cannot exist unless its membership consists of more than one person, it is equally true that a group cannot exist without some minimal structure and commonly held purpose or goals. The leader's task is first and foremost to provide for the health of the group (i.e., maintenance function) and facilitate the group's movement toward its goals (i.e., task function). Specifically, the group leader is responsible for *setting standards, creating a facilitative atmosphere, and promoting effective communications.*

Setting Standards. Like any social situation, a group functions with a set of norms, roles, and goals. The leader is responsible for identifying the operating norms (rules of conduct) and making these clearly known to all members. While the specific rules will vary from group to group, depending upon group composition, setting, and task, one rule or norm should remain constant and that is, that the group exists to serve a purpose, or achieve a goal, while meeting the unique needs of its members. Group members need to be encouraged to articulate their own particular hopes and aspirations; and these should be compared to the formally expressed intent of the group. Laying individual agendas on the table so that they may be dealt with directly is essential for any group to function effectively.

Creating a Facilitative Environment. In order for the group to benefit from the numbers and talents of its membership, the atmosphere must be one that promotes a sense of trust among the members. In order for individuals to be willing to share their feelings, ideas, or resources with another, they must feel that the other will not only appreciate this sharing but will be supportive of them when such support is needed. The group leader needs to establish this atmosphere of *support, trust, mutual respect, and concern* by being the model of such open, trusting, supportive interaction.

Promoting Effective Communication. In addition to providing an environment and set of norms that encourage interaction, the leader should provide direction (via instruction or modeling) as to how to communicate effectively within the group. Individuals should be made aware that all self-disclosure needs to be relevant to the current state of the group. Rather than simply rambling about oneself or one's legacy, an individual might disclose the "here and now" effect the group may be having upon him/her, or how he/she feels he/she is impacting the group. Similarly, in responding to another, a group member should be "instructed" (directly by the leader or as modeled by the leader) to be *active* and responsive to the content and affect expressed in the messages. Finally, the leader needs to promote facilitative confrontation by encouraging others to confront themselves during periods of passive observation or silence, or even when they find themselves taking the posture of the underminer. Adequate and facilitative confrontation is a basic staple of the fully functioning group, and the leader provides the model that will be followed in this potentially productive process.

A good group leader understands the principles of group process and is sensitive to changes in the tone of a group and alterations in the interpersonal style of each of its participants. In addition to self-awareness and calm acceptance of the emotional and intellectual onslaughts that must be endured, knowledge of the principles of group selection and group evolution are vital to the leader's goal of making the group a worthwhile experience for its members.

Composition of a Group

Determining what types of individuals are desirable for a particular group is an important decision for the leader. The criteria for inclusion of individuals in a group vary, depending upon such factors as the group's overall purpose, the specific goals of each member, and the methodology employed by the leader or co-leaders.

Boenheim and his associates developed a specific set of criteria for exclusion or inclusion when setting up a pilot psychotherapy group with adolescents:

> It took considerable time to select the membership of a pilot group of girls and boys. We knew from our experience with adult groups that proper selection...is the main safeguard against failure from the very start. We were, therefore, determined not to overburden our difficult task by accepting cases of widely different intelligence, social status, and upbringing. I did not include psychotics or delinquents, but concentrated on girls and boys who had difficulties in mixing with members of their own and the opposite sex, who were shy, introverted, self-conscious or had problems with their parents and siblings and felt generally unhappy (Boenheim, 1957, p. 400).

Yalom, a noted expert in group psychotherapy, indicates that poor candidates for intensive group therapy include sociopaths, organically brain-damaged persons, the suicidal, addicted individuals, the acutely psychotic, paranoid persons, the extremely self-centered, and the hypochondriacal. He offers a number of reasons why these categories of individuals should be excluded.

> These patients seem destined to fail because of their inability to participate in the primary task of the group; they soon construct an interpersonal role which proves to be detrimental to themselves as well as to the group (Yalom, 1975, p. 158).

However, leadership roles in groups of this type are not required of most workers unless they elect to specialize and have acquired advanced training.

The ordinary worker is more likely to be involved in a leadership role in the following types of groups:

1. Brief family counseling
2. Supervision groups
3. Community groups
4. Short-term patient groups or meetings

In these cases, the leader is often presented with a ready-made group. One may be asked to see a client's family, a group of trainees, or several community members, or be requested to hold a morning meeting with clients in a crisis unit. Such clients may be psychotics, psychoneurotics, addicts, or a mixed group. There is little choice for the leader in the matter of group composition.

However, knowledge of group composition is essential for dealing with previously formed groups and for the process of identifying clients who will be difficult to handle. For example, if one is scheduled to be a co-leader of a group of patients on a short-term psychiatric unit made up of eight verbal neurotics, a seriously brain-damaged, elderly female suffering from the results of tertiary syphilis, and a male catatonic schizophrenic, one must take the makeup of the group into account before the first meeting.

In this instance, it can be expected that the brain-damaged individual will have problems comprehending what is taking place, or have difficulty with self-control. Therefore, someone may be seated next to her to assist her as needed. The catatonic will be uncommunicative, but will probably be aware of what is occurring and may be brought into the discussion by getting the other patients to talk about how they're dealing with him. The patient is unlikely to respond to such a discussion, but he probably is listening, and this may become evident later when he begins to communicate verbally with the group or a staff member.

Here are several signs that may indicate that an individual may cause difficulty in a group, drop out, or contribute to the failure of the group.

1. The individual who is significantly different from other members in terms of age, background, needs, intelligence, or occupation
2. One who is extremely withdrawn
3. The person who is very self-centered and talkative
4. The grossly disturbed participant in a group that is comprised of persons who are reasonably well oriented to reality
5. The person on the edge of a crisis just prior to or during the initial stage of the group

6. The participant who tends toward immediate, unrealistic self-disclosure early in the group
7. The person who fails to appear at several group meetings

It should be emphasized that a group with one or more of these types of individuals need not fail if the leader is aware of their methods of interacting and has sufficient skill to deal with their impact. An example may be seen in the self-centered and talkative individual, who may be effectively cut off, redirected, or silenced by group reaction.

If the efforts to get persons involved are having their desired effects, the participants should begin to see improvement in their own performance or in that of other group members. This will tend to increase confidence in the future, build feelings of acceptance, and even develop pride in the group.

Life of a Group

Groups differ in content, rates of progress, and goals they seek and are able to achieve. Despite this variance, most groups proceed through similar stages if they survive over a sufficient period of time. These stages can be broadly classified as (1) exploration and orientation, (2) conflict and flight, (3) integration, (4) working alliance, and (5) termination.

During the initial stage of *exploration and orientation*, members normally experience anxiety over their involvement in the group and the outcome they hope for. During this period, people introduce themselves; begin to formulate rules for interaction; and, often at the urging of a more outspoken member, establish social roles for interaction. Common ground is sought, as well as recognition from the group leader. During this time the group may tend to be philosophical and intellectual, or it may spend a good deal of time chatting about issues of no great consequence.

The second stage centers around *conflict* as members begin to reveal their characteristic patterns of dealing with others and form subgroups. Confrontations between members, between member subgroups, and between members and the group leader usually take place. The leader can expect to be put on the spot by some of the group members at this stage, particularly by those who are having trouble with self-assertion and dependency, but who have started experimenting with aggressive techniques to ward off their fears of being reliant on others. In this phase, the problem members reveal themselves and must be dealt with if the group is to last. This category of difficult group members will include people who are extremely withdrawn, dramatic but resistant, very talkative, and those who attempt to qualify as "the leader's helper."

Such participants may be handled in a number of ways:

1. Extremely withdrawn
   a. Focus on this person with a question or a comment designed to elicit from him or her some opinion on the topic under discussion.
   b. Ask the group what it thinks about members who remain silent during the session.
   c. Recognize the member's unexpressed feelings about a topic being commented on by others in the group. ("John, you seem to agree with what Bill is saying.")
2. Dramatic but resistant
   a. This individual often asks for assistance, but rejects help offered by the group. The group may then show frustration, perhaps shared by the leader, and a general feeling of hopelessness may result. This may be counteracted by focusing on the hidden agenda in the rejector's dramatic comment. "Jill, you say that you have problems in relating to others, but when suggestions are made they never seem to be what you're looking for. Maybe this pattern of requesting and rejecting help is one we need to focus on, rather than the difficulties you perceive."
   b. Another way to deal with the person who has problems that no members of the group can understand or help with is to offer agreement. "I don't think we can help you with the problem you've brought up. You're right. It's no use."
3. Very talkative
   a. Redirect member's focus.
   b. Interrupt and return to task.
   c. Confront in terms of their potential contributions and strengths, as well as the deleterious effects of their talkativeness.
   d. Ignore and extinguish the talkativeness, through failure to recognize or affirm.
4. "Leader's helper"
   a. The need to ally with the leader can spring from a variety of motives. A common technique in dealing with such an individual is to encourage recognition of his or her difficulties.
   b. When the leader's helper objects that help is not needed, the group may be asked to comment on such a display of self-sufficiency; or the leader may point this out by remarking, "Sam, you don't seem to have the same difficulties as others in the group."

Often the extent to which the members demonstrate these troublesome behaviors is so great that it creates a generalized desire among the group members to avoid group interaction. Such a "flight or avoidance" tendency often exhibits itself in a number of ways. Groups that find they sit in the same places, chat about the same things, do the same activities, and in general appear to be a ritualized, inflexible entity may be demonstrating the symptoms of group flight. Similarly, groups that attempt to focus on one or another individual, or rehash old problems or relive old victories, thus avoiding the here and now may again be demonstrating a generalized conflict behavior. Under these conditions, the leader needs to not only confront the group members about the apparent generalized sense of conflict and the need for such flight behavior, but also establish, as the group's immediate goal, the identification and reduction of the source of this conflict, and the redevelopment of the trusting, supportive climate needed for positive group interaction.

When the conflict stage is passed, the group enters a phase of togetherness, in which *integration* takes place and members feel comfortable with each other. Individuals show concern for others and demonstrate a need to be liked by the whole group.

This integrated stage leads to a fourth one, in which a working alliance is formed between the members. At this point communication opens up, with some members functioning as discussion leaders in addition to their roles as participants in need of help. A block to self-disclosure that can develop at this stage is the occurrence of meetings and discussions outside of the group, perhaps including several members. The fringe group must be encouraged to confine its discussions to the parent group.

The fifth and final stage is *termination*, which can take several forms. The group may terminate as a whole, or one member may do so. An individual may terminate at an appropriate juncture, as when he feels progress has been sufficient for his needs, or he may do so prematurely. If the leader thinks termination is premature, the member may be asked to discuss it in a separate meeting or the question may be brought up in the group. If the termination comes at an appropriate time, it may be pointed out that the experience should be accepted as a normal phenomenon, but one that is intended to make future interactions more satisfactory to all concerned.

Basic Techniques and Principles in Group Work

In learning how to work with groups, as in training to deal therapeutically with individuals, there are numerous techniques and principles that can be mastered to improve results. Some are applicable to short-term, task-oriented groups as well as to therapy groups.

Handling practical matters. In the beginning, the leader must ensure that arrangements for the group meeting place are complete. In the first meeting, procedures, length of the group meetings, and number of sessions planned should be discussed, as well as how many members will be desirable or necessary. Policy concerning the admission of new members should also be discussed.

Group and individual goals must be taken into account simultaneously.

While intervening to ensure that a member is not left out of group discussion, it is essential to avoid excessive concern for individual members, as this can lead to loss of control.

One must determine what each person wants to get out of the group. Through observation and direct inquiry, the leader should find out what each member wants from the group experience, for if an individual feels support is lacking, he or she may drop out early in the group's evolution.

If selection has been made correctly, the leader should not have difficulty eliciting and emphasizing group commonalities. Unless a group member feels that he or she possesses something in common with others, continued participation may be thought useless.

Group unity is necessary if the group is to have an impact on each participant's behavior. A group can set standards of behavior and provide a model of how interpersonal relations can be effectively conducted and interpersonal problems successfully resolved. However, before this occurs, the participant must be convinced of the group's importance and of the trustworthiness of its members.

Uncovering and communicating group and individual agendas is a function of the leader. Through direct interpretation, question, and confrontation, or by eliciting comments from the group, the leader should uncover hidden agendas, expose power struggles, and explain the reasons for the apathy, hostility, or talkativeness of particular individuals, or why others are transmitting nonverbal messages. A technique to reveal a hidden agenda when members persist in talking about peripheral topics may be in the form of a comment, as follows: "We've been sitting here for half an hour talking about _____. I wonder why we are doing this. Is there something we all are avoiding?" As the group progresses, the leader will be less directive when a hidden agenda is detected. A comment such as, "I wonder what's going on here now?" will convey the message to the members. Occasionally the leader may prefer to wait until a group member intervenes.

The pace of the group is dependent upon each member's ability to progress toward the group goal. In the selection process, the leader tries to avoid gathering members who are widely divergent in their needs, intelligence, or interests. Despite such efforts, the differences between members are often accentuated in the group. It is the job of the leader to ensure that such differences as those, for example, in individual members' abilities to reveal personal secrets or admit mistakes do not result in uneven progress within the group.

An essential function of the leader is to facilitate communication. By reflecting a question or occasionally remaining silent when asked to respond, the leader will encourage members to be less dependent and to interact with others in the group. Particularly in the group's initial stages, the leader must set the tone, perhaps by asking the group to respond to the question, or by redirecting a member's question onto another member who appears to be uninvolved.

The manner in which a group responds is just as important as what it says. The content of the group's exchange is critical, but how its messages are sent and received is equally important. If a member raises an issue that brings an emotional response from the group, this must be noted and discussed. "I noticed that when Sherry brought up the topic of suicide, everyone really got upset. What do you think that was all about?"

The group should focus its attention on interactions taking place now. While historical material is useful in examining a member's problems and in determining how he or she is learning from the group, interpersonal relations within the group yield more pertinent data and enliven group discussion.

Summary

Groups offer their members the opportunity to let off steam, acquire knowledge and skills for professional use, learn how others interact or do their jobs, gain social support, and, in general, learn how to work through problems that cannot be solved alone.

When the health professional has mastered the principles of group process through work and study, expertise as a group leader will come with experience in that role. Mental health workers, physician's assistants, licensed practical nurses, college students, assistant caseworkers, correctional counselors, and other human service personnel and trainees are currently successfully involved in group work as co-leaders in various settings.

It should be emphasized that skill in working with groups is more and more a necessity for the human service worker, and, to meet this responsibility successfully, thorough training in group dynamics and group leadership is required.

10 / *report writing and referrals*

Reports are usually written with two purposes in mind: to establish a printed record for future reference, and to communicate up-to-date information on a particular case. To be useful, a report should be clear, concise, and complete. These objectives are easily grasped, but their achievement requires concentrated effort. Poor psychological, psychiatric, and social work reports are commonplace. Vagueness, poor organization, unnecessary jargon, and failure to substantiate inferential comments are the most common weaknesses in many reports. Learning how to write a useful, well-reasoned report is a skill that some professionals and paraprofessionals never acquire, despite intensive training in other aspects of their work.

The development of a clear and logical report-writing style requires much time and effort in which the following factors must be recognized:

1. The audience for which the report is intended
2. The questions to be asked to determine material that will form the descriptive information and that will substantiate the inferential material
3. The plan to be used to recognize and integrate data

Audience

"For whom is the report intended?" is the first question that confronts the writer. For example, a report written exclusively for school teachers probably would not present enough material on a client's psychodynamics to be satisfactory in the judgment of a psychologist or a psychiatrist assigned to a mental health unit. Similarly, a report developed for a mental health worker conducting psychotherapy should emphasize current environmental and interpersonal factors in the client's life in order to facilitate concentration by the worker on returning the client to the community promptly. A report that failed to emphasize such elements would be useless.

Only by knowing the intended audience can the writer determine the emphasis and technical level of a report—when to include or exclude certain information, and how best to present various data. Inasmuch as terminology is useful only to the extent that it is understandable, the writer must exercise care when including it in the report. Even when the report is intended for use by mental health workers, psychological and psychiatric terminology lacks the preciseness common to older sciences such as physics or biology.

Terminology. In most sciences, terminology is normally specific, in that definitions are both limited and direct and generally agreed upon. For example, when an investigator speaks of the process of *ablation*, it can be expected that other scientists will understand this to refer to a surgical procedure involving excision or amputation of a part of the body. Even the most basic terminology is used with care by physical scientists, who are mindful even of alternative meanings of terms when they are applied by professionals in allied fields. The term "ablation," for example, has other meanings when applied in other fields, as when an aerospace specialist uses it to refer to the dissipation of heat generated by atmospheric friction.

The temptation to resort to technical jargon can be irresistible. Frequently, the meaning given a term by one group of psychologists is not acceptable to another segment of professionals. Such terms as "borderline," "latent homosexual," or even the commonly used label "passive-aggressive" do not have meanings generally acceptable to most mental health professionals.

When terms fail to convey accurate information on which to base treatment decisions, this leads to confusion in reports of client diagnosis. Jargon is to be avoided unless it is appropriate for the audience for whom the report is intended. Unfortunately, too often novices sprinkle their reports with technical terms in an effort to appear professional—a technique inadvertently taught in many instances by their supervisors.

Questions to Be Asked

Just as it is important to know the intended audience for a report, familiarity with the questions to which the report is to be directed is essential. Too often reports are written in response to vague questions or with no clear comprehension of the specific questions being asked, resulting in broad generalizations and unsound conclusions or recommendations. This can be prevented by responding to a general inquiry with further questions to determine more precisely what information is being sought.

The following are a few examples of questions designed to clarify general inquiries:

I'd like to know in a report just how the client is doing?
In what respect?
Please give me a general report on how _____ is coming along.
What kinds of things are you specifically interested in knowing?

These questions may be followed by others until the writer has acquired sufficient information to guide him or her in the preparation of an outline and, eventually, a complete report.

Before examining how a typical mental health report is organized, a few additional errors to be avoided should be noted.

Common Errors in Report Writing

Most of the difficulties or problems encountered in the process of preparing a useful report relate to three broad questions that arise as the report is developed:

1. What information do I need to include?
2. How do I present a balanced picture of the person?
3. To what extent do I present inferences and theories as to why and how the client is behaving?

What Information to Include. When the question asked relates to the client's intelligence, information from interviews and psychological testing will be used to determine actual talents and deficits, including those capabilities that may be tapped in the future. These should deal in detail with such factors as the client's abilities and shortcomings in abstract reasoning, memory (long- and short-term), arithmetical skills, general fund of information, common sense, and visual-motor skills. Also, there should be coverage of factors that indirectly affect intelligence, including personality functioning, occupational and educational history, vocational aspirations, and interpersonal relations.

For example, if a middle-aged male is termed "above average," the following additional questions would aim to show how his intelligence is used and is involved in other areas:

Personality Functioning. Since he is above average in intelligence, does he tend to use intellectualism as a defense? That is, does he evade others and his own emotions by rationalizing and denying the presence of any reaction, even in emotionally charged situations?

Occupational and Educational History. Does his education and job experience show him to be an overachiever or an underachiever, or do these accord with his current intellectual abilities?

Vocational Aspirations. Do his future goals appear realistic in terms of his intellectual capability?

Interpersonal Relations. Do his interactions with his peers and the reporter seem compatible with the level of intellect reflected in observation and testing, or does he seem to wish to appear above or below this level?

In this example we have seen that while one area is normally emphasized in a report, other areas should receive some attention in order to give a complete picture. Various aspects of the whole person, as well as elements in the client's environment that intensify or that may help to alleviate a problem, should be covered in some degree when responding to specific questions about an individual's intellect or personality.

This is not to suggest that the report should provide a lengthy, detailed coverage of all areas, but rather that the client should not be compartmentalized artificially. Personality affects intelligence even as intelligence affects personality. Thus, when the report relates to the question of referral, a picture of the whole person is desirable. This is particularly important when the question concerns pathology or deviant behavior potential.

A Balanced Picture. A common error made in report preparation is excessive emphasis on the pathological or negative aspects of the client's personality and environment. Many, perhaps most, reports tend to dwell on what is wrong with clients, their families, and interpersonal environments, with little mention of the positive factors in the client's person or environment. It is as if psychologists, social workers, and psychiatrists prefer to see the worst and to tell sad stories about their clients. This tendency is counteracted to some degree by the current movement to explore and respond to the client's assets and environmental support systems, rather than to focus on pathological considerations. However, care should be taken not to delete essential pathological information in the effort to accent positive factors.

An illustration may be seen in the case of a twenty-one-year-old female secretary admitted to an emergency inpatient unit after abusing others in her office verbally and physically. Following a week's stay in the unit, a report was requested concerning her potential future behavior. Did the staff feel she would act out and become abusive again if released? The staff report emphasized the following negative factors:

Client still disoriented after one week
Uncooperative with staff members

Mother divorced when client was six years old
Job very stressful

The write-up failed to give adequate attention to the following positive factors:

Client manifested no new outbursts while on unit
Abusive episode was the *first* recorded and appeared suddenly (a good prognostic indicator)
Client had functioned well in her occupation up to the point of the episode
Relationship with mother was good
Two brothers who lived in area showed active desire to become involved in supportive work with client
Client had begun to verbalize feelings more rationally and expressed interest in returning to work
Client expressed willingness to enter group therapy

Obviously, workers should not treat the report as an opportunity for displaying expertise in their descriptions of disease and symptomatology, but should note, for example, the absence of further deterioration and similar positive factors.

Inferences and Theories. Another common error in report writing is facile theorizing by the worker. Some reporters tend to weave theories out of thin air and unobservable constructs, while others fail to integrate their material; data are presented as a jumble of disconnected facts, so that the reader cannot get a clear total picture or follow main threads in the report. A theory of personality is basic to a cohesive picture, and without it a good report cannot be made. Workers are obligated to substantiate claims made in their reports, and this requires some knowledge of personality theory—how and why individuals act as they do.

Presenting several inferences based on one's previous experience and training normally is no problem. Also, it may be useful for the reporter to offer some behavioral theory *after* facts and illustrative observations have been presented. When guesses based solely on intuition are made, the report fails to reflect informed and well-reasoned observation. It is possible to find a happy medium between listing disparate facts and weaving elaborate and unfounded theories, but this requires acute observation and sensitive interpretation.

Organizing a Report

There is no one correct way to organize a mental health report. The form will vary from writer to writer, depending on the questions asked, the audience for which it is intended, and the depth of information that is required.

As we have noted in chapter 2, a historical interview or mental status report can be quite lengthy. However, the format for the write-up becomes less circumscribed outside the standard historical or in-depth intake session. Style normally is not specified when reports on particular questions are requested. Since the worker's findings and impressions are essentially what is sought, the approach need only be logical, coherent, and reasonably complete.

Table 10.1 presents a brief outline for a typical psychological report in response to a specific question about a client's status.

Identifying Data. In brief reports designed to answer specific questions, identifying data are kept to a minimum. A general rule is to provide just enough information to allow the agent requesting the report and the writer to differentiate between the subject of the report and other clients. Data included are normally classed under the following headings:

Name	Date
Age	Person who prepared
	report
Sex	Agency and address of
	reporter

Table 10.1 Psychological Report Outline—A Sample

Identifying Data
Sources of Information
Recent Behavior and Physical Appearance
    (Behavior and appearance during interview, on hospital ward, in day
    hospital...)
Pertinent Historical Data
Medical and Intellectual Status
Personality
    (Manner in which person deals with world, interests, drives...)
Social
    (Relations with others, style of interacting with interviewer, type of
    environment person comes from and what it has to offer patient upon
    return...)
Integration of Data
    (Summary and impressions)
Diagnosis—optional
    (Usually followed by a description of person, to rule out misunderstandings
    in this area)
Prognosis
Recommendations

Race Reason for report
Address Referral questions

Sources. The reporter should next indicate the sources of the information, since this will have a bearing on the validity of the impressions received. If many sources are used or there has been lengthy contact with the client, the accuracy of the material will tend to be greater than if the report was based on a brief contact with the client alone.
 Sources might include the following:

 Interview with client (duration of contact and in what capacity should be noted)
 Records (hospital, school, etc.)
 Psychological tests
 Neurological or lab tests
 Contacts with family, friends, employer, nursing staff, and the like

Whenever possible, reference should be made to the particular source that provided items of information, whether from the client alone, records, family, and so on.

Recent Behavior. In this section, the client's physical appearance and behavior during the most recent contacts are covered in order to give the reader a reasonably clear impression of how the client appeared to the writer in their most recent contact. It may also provide clues as to how the client felt during the interview: for example, hostile, apathetic, depressed, anxious. A brief paragraph or two will usually suffice.

Pertinent History. While extensive historical material has no place in a brief psychological report, such information spontaneously offered by the client in a reality-oriented session occasionally relates to the problem at hand. In some instances, the reporter may feel there are elements in the client's past that have direct bearing on the information being given, for example, past hospitalizations or pathological episodes.

Medical and Intellectual Assessment. Two areas that may receive a great deal of attention are those concerned with the client's physical health and intellectual status. The degree to which these sections are emphasized is variable, depending on a number of factors.
 If a client's actual physical health or subjective assessment of his or her own medical well-being is relevant to the issues, of course it should be noted in reports. If physical condition is not an issue, there is no need for its inclusion or coverage in a brief report.
 However, most reports discuss intelligence. The amount of attention it

receives will vary and will naturally be greater in instances in which this information is specifically requested. In cases in which an intellectual assessment is not directly requested, it may be presented only in terms of its impact on the client's personality status.

Personality Dynamics.   As might be expected, personality dynamics is of great importance in most psychiatric and psychological reports. This reflects the fact that most psychologists, psychiatric social workers, psychiatrists, and mental health workers feel their expertise lies in this area, and questions about personality are, therefore, common. This section of the report frequently presents a detailed picture of the client's emotional problems and personality strengths, but it may also contain a great deal of useless jargon. Most experienced workers who have some knowledge of personality theory will find this section of the report within their competence. Avoidance of jargon can often help to make a report more practical and useful than one prepared in the more traditional professional style.

Typical questions that may be covered under the personality dynamics heading are as follows:

How does the client generally view his or her person? Low self-image? The world? Threatening, happy, bland?

What kinds of roles and interpersonal images does the client tend to foster?

What types and degrees of stress disturb the client?

What conflicts does the client find most disturbing?

How does the client deal with frustration, aggression, withdrawal, displacement?

How well do strategies of dealing with frustration and conflict succeed?

What are the client's greatest personal difficulties? How serious are they?

What personal assets are strong (maturity, control of gratification, flexibility, sense of humor, self-control, intelligence, persistence, etc.)?

Social.   Emphasis on the client's preferred interpersonal roles is here extended by inquiry into the environment. This will consist of interviews with the client's friends coupled with the client's responses to questions about friends and family, including how well or poorly interactions develop. This has been an area of strong concentration by social workers for many years. Fortunately, psychiatrists and psychologists today are moving away from exclusive concern with intrapsychic factors and, instead, are turning to social areas to seek help from others in the client's environment. Awareness of the client's world helps to avoid the trap of seeing an individual as a mere pathological entity.

Summarization. Once groundwork has been completed, material can be integrated and summarized. This portion of the report thus consists of a brief answer to the principal question being explored. A diagnosis may be offered, if appropriate. This may be followed by a prognosis indicating possible outcome of treatment.

Finally, any recommendations the writer wishes to make may be listed; these would be both practical and specific. They may vary from a suggestion that chemotherapy be continued to a recommendation for further evaluation by psychological testing, interviews, neurological scans, and so on.

Evaluating and Making a Referral

In some instances, a report will contain a referral for treatment; in others, the report is issued in response to a referral for evaluation or treatment. The responsibility for the preparation of such referrals, evaluations, or recommendations often falls to the worker, who must first determine whether the referral question is clear. If it is not, more information from the source of the referral is required. The next step is to determine whether the questions being asked are within the scope of the worker's competence. Refusal of a referral because of lack of sufficient skill or experience should not be seen as a fault or shortcoming in the worker. Rather, it would be a serious error— as well as unethical—to accept a referral that was beyond the capability or competence of the worker. When there is doubt, the supervisor or unit director should be consulted. This consultation will often bring helpful advice on how to handle the problem, in effect, an increment to the worker's training and a broadening of his or her experience. A typical instance might be one in which a mental health worker's first referral of a depressed person is accepted with the understanding that a psychiatrist, psychologist, or psychiatric social worker will supervise the therapeutic work.

The final point to make on receiving a referral concerns the way in which the material received from the referring agent should be viewed. This information is frequently useful, but at times can be very misleading. It must be recognized that while the source of the referral is not intent on misleading anyone, the information is affected by another's bias. This requires a degree of healthy skepticism when evaluating the information to prevent being unduly influenced by the referring agent's perspective. Since the need for a fresh viewpoint or opinion is often the reason for a request for referral, there need be no reluctance to form an independent judgment.

The time of a referral is an important consideration. Some professionals delay too long before deciding to secure a psychiatric or psychological assessment of the client. This is likely to be especially true in cases of persistently depressive and chronically anxious office patients.

In some cases medical doctors or physician's associates feel they are abdicating responsibility if they send someone for an evaluation by a mental health professional. Their attitude may be: "We can handle it here; the individual is just upset a lot of the time because of fear or uncertainty." In fact, one of the key responsibilities of the line medical professional is to determine when further information is needed; thus, screening is one of their functions. For example in the case of a cancer patient, if, after support and chemotherapy are administered in general practice or at the medical clinic, the client continues to be depressed or anxious, a referral for psychological testing or assessment is indicated.

Another consideration that may discourage medical personnel from making a referral is client resistance to psychological or psychiatric evaluation. The physician may rationalize: "I don't like to suggest a referral to a psychiatrist, psychologist, or clinic because I'll get a negative response from the patient. 'Do you think I'm nuts, doc?' "

While such concern is understandable, the fear is often unrealistic. Many clients respond with relief and renewed hope for a solution to their problem; others may question the decision but agree when assured it's in their best interest.

The following illustration is an example of how a negative response by a depressed adult male might be handled:

> *Client:* "You think I'm nuts because I'm so blue all the time. Is that why you're referring me to a shrink?"
> *Physician:* "No, I don't think you're 'nuts,' Mr._____. A psychiatrist is just another medical specialist, like a radiologist. And just as I would refer you to a radiologist if you were in need of an x-ray, I'm referring you to a psychiatrist to see what he thinks about your being down most of the time. He's an expert in analyzing all types of depression and will be able to give us some advice on how to deal with it."

In this instance, as in many similar cases, a prompt referral is the best means of providing the client with effective treatment.

Summary

The ability to write a good report is the result of careful attention and hard work. Clear, concise, and complete reports that are tailored to the questions asked must be prepared with an awareness of the report's goal and its intended audience.

A final point should be made regarding the *confidentiality* of written reports. Increasingly, clients are exercising their right of access to reports that are kept on file in schools, hospitals, and clinics. The writer should realize this fact before developing a report.

In addition, while clergymen, physicians, and lawyers are not subject to subpoena with regard to the notes they make during interviews with clients, most allied health professionals are. Although such circumstances are rare, they occur often enough to make noting them here appropriate.

11 / *the consulting process*

If the only task of human service professionals were to diagnose and treat clients, the following discussion would be unnecessary. Knowledge about providing *direct service* to the client is most important, but it is just one area with which the human service worker must be concerned.

In addition to assuming a role as diagnostician and remediator, human service workers are often called upon to provide guidance and direction to other professionals who are similarly involved with the client. In the role of *consultant* human service personnel not only indirectly serve the client (by providing assistance to another person responsible for the care and treatment of the client), but also help to expand the effects of their interventions by impacting the extrapersonal factors supporting the client's problem. Further, in line with our emphasis upon seeking to provide services that have a preventative nature, consultation proves quite effective.

The role of a consultant is a difficult role to master. The following chapter attempts to outline the role and duties of the *consultant* and his or her client, the *consultee*, in order to increase the effectiveness of the human service worker, who is often called to play the roles of both consultant and consultee.

What Is Consultation?

The terms "consultation" and "consultant" have recently come in vogue. As a result, quite a number of varied and unrelated acts and job descriptions have become grouped under the rubric of consultation. The current discussion will not provide an elaborate discussion of the various models and schools of thought on the nature of consultation, but will provide an eclectic orientation to the issue of mental health consultation. The reader interested in a more detailed presentation of the history and theoretical foundations of mental health consultation is referred to the presentation of Meyers, Parsons, and Martin (1979).

A starting point for defining consultation is to note that it is a helping relationship. Consultation is a *problem-solving* process that occurs between two or more professionals. It is characteristically a voluntary relationship in which a current work problem of the consultee is the focus of the collaborative problem solving of both the consultant and consultee. In addition to resolving the current work problem, consultation that is effective will also assist the consultee in developing those skills and attitudes needed to handle future problems more effectively.

Like other helping relationships (e.g., therapy, counseling), consultation involves facilitative communication and interpersonal skills. Consultation, however, differs from these other forms of helping in a number of significant ways.

A Triadic Relationship. Consultation, as defined within the text, involves the interaction of a professional help-giver (the consultant) and a help-seeker (the consultee) who is responsible for the welfare of another person (client). Thus, a social worker, working as a consultant, may be asked to provide a psychiatric nurse (the consultee) with diagnostic information and recommendations for intervention with an alcoholic client.

Consultation, as seen in the example, involves at least a triadic relationship and in this respect is unlike the more typical dyad of the counseling interchange. With its focus on impacting the client, by way of effecting change in the consultee, consultation is by definition an indirect service delivery model.

Interaction of Colleagues. Gerald Caplan (1970) noted that consultation should be a nonhierarchical relationship. In this sense, consultation involves two or more professionals who each bring to the interaction some unique expertise that bears on the analysis and intervention of the problem at hand. While expertise is situation and participant specific, it can be generally stated that the consultant provides expertise in the principles and practice applicable to the remediation of the specific problem under investigation; whereas the consultee (the individual contracting for consultation assistance, for example, a therapist or agency) possesses greater knowledge of and familiarity with the circumstances and characteristics surrounding the client and the problem.

The collegial nature of consultation demands that the responsibility for problem resolution be shared mutually by consultant and consultee. Thus, the consultant must not enter the relationship as the "savior" or "grand problem solver," but rather as one who can facilitate the consultee's mobilization of his/her own resources for the resolution of the problem at hand.

Consultee May Reject Advice.   One of the unique characteristics of consultation is that not only is the consultee viewed as a colleague in the problem resolution, but the consultant is clear that the consultee may accept or reject the consultant's recommendations at any time. Further, the relationship between the consultant and consultee should be voluntary and, as such, the consultee can terminate the relationship at any time.

Focus on Prevention as Well as Remediation.   One of the most important goals of consultation is not only to help solve the current work problem of the help-seeker, but also to assist the help-seeker to profit from the experience in such a way that future problems may be handled more sensitively and skillfully. Thus, when a clinical case worker (the consultee) requests assistance from a psychiatrist (the consultant) with interviewing a difficult client, not only will the recommendations help with this specific case, but should increase the consultee's interview skills and competence in dealing with future cases.

This educational focus of consultation provides a basis from which the consultant may impact not only the original client, but similar clients who are under the care of the consultee. It is through the potential for such educational ripple effects that consultation appears to serve the preventive goals that have previously been depicted as essential to the human service arena (see introduction). As a preventive service, consultation attempts to foster the development of skills and procedures in the consultee that not only ameliorate the client's problem, but can be used to reduce the impact or duration of similar problems in the future. Further, such consultation intervention attempts to create changes in those extrapersonal factors (e.g., the consultee, the client's organization) that contribute to the development of client problems, thus helping to *prevent* similar problems in the future.

Forms of Services Rendered

During the last ten to fifteen years a growing number of professionals have written about the content and process of consultation. One immediate result of this increased attention is that a variety of methods and approaches have been developed. Consultation, for example, has been presented from varied orientations and theoretical perspectives (Platt and Wicks, 1979), as behavioral modification (Bergen, 1977); mental health focus (Caplan, 1970); organizational development (Bennis, 1969); and educational or school orientation (Meyers, Parsons, and Martin, 1979).

Often writers on consultation attempt to contrast consultation with various forms of direct service delivery (e.g., therapy, counseling). While it is true that many practices do *directly* involve the client (e.g., individual counseling), such activity does not exclude indirect services. Most of the services we provide involve some element of direct service and indirect service to the client. The worker who, after counseling a young client regarding his inability to be assertive with his peers, provides feedback and recommendations to the client's parents, is not only potentially impacting the client via his/her direct intervention (i.e., counseling), but may also be indirectly impacting the client by providing therapeutic feedback and recommendations to the client's parents.

Using this continuum of direct-indirect service delivery as a basis, Meyers, Parsons, and Martin (1979) provided a framework for conceptualizing consultation. This framework depicts four broad categories of service: direct service to the client, indirect service to the client, direct service to the consultee, and service to the system/organization. Each of these categories is briefly described below.

Direct Service to the Client. Very often human service workers, in an attempt to be cost effective, meet a client and attempt to gather all of the diagnostic material by themselves. Further, they often take full responsibility for the intervention and remediation of the client's problem.

Workers operating from a consultation orientation also attempt to gather diagnostic material through direct interview or testing. In addition, however, they have the consultee (e.g., the client's teacher, supervisor, parent, family physician) gather observational data and work artifacts (e.g., school papers, memos), which are then included in the diagnostic process. Similarly, operating within a consultation framework, they attempt to involve any significant others in the client's life into the remediation and treatment. Therefore, typical procedures in a consultation approach involving direct services to the client are having the client's teacher run behavior modification programs, working with the parents as co-therapist, or employing the client's middle line manager as skill trainer.

Indirect Service to the Client. Most typically, consultation is viewed as a process wherein the consultant fails to have direct contact with the client. However, consultation can be viewed more positively as a process wherein the service is indirectly provided to the client using the *consultee* as principal agent. The services rendered through this form of consultation directly impact the "caretakers" of the client. Thus, discussion is set up with the client's teachers, peers, co-workers, supervisors, or allied health professionals, and they (the consultees) implement the intervention strategies. An example of such consultation occurs when a community health nurse (the consultant) provides a program of physical therapy to be implemented by a client's spouse (the consultee) as part of a home care program.

Direct Service to the Consultee. Often the nature of the client's presenting problem implies that a significant factor in the maintenance and creation of the difficulty is the attitude, feelings, or actions of the consultee. One example is reflected in the case of a black worker who is nonproductive and openly hostile at work and who is supervised by an elderly man who refers to all his workers as "boys." In this type of situation, providing service directly to the consultee (i.e., supervisor) appears to be the most efficient means of intervention. Thus, rather than attempting to modify the client's behavior, the focus is on changing the consultee's behavior, attitudes, and/or feelings. Such a change would not only impact the client, but all future clients coming under the care of that consultee.

Service to the System/Organization.   Often a consultant is asked to provide service to an organization or system. Again, while the request might focus on improving communications within the system, adjusting the social system to improve productivity, or modifying the administrative or managerial aspects of an organization, ultimately the impact of the consultation will be on the improved functioning of the organization's members and thus may serve a preventive service. That is, by helping to create a more positive, productive, and supportive environment, the consultant is removing many of those stressors and environmental conditions that create or aggravate mental health problems. As such, intervention at the system level appears to be one of the most cost-efficient approaches to providing mental health services to all those involved with the organization.

The bias of the authors of this text is that the true preventive value and potential of consultation is best served when the consultant can effect change at the broadest level. As such, whenever possible, attempting to provide service to the system should be considered as the level of choice. Further, even when the consultant is requested to provide services directly to a client, he/she should attempt to impact both the consultee and the system at large. For example, a psychologist who received repeated requests from a teacher for psychological testing of "disturbed children," would increase the impact of his/her services if, in providing feedback to the consultee (i.e., the teacher), he/she also provided a method for valid screening and early detection of high risk children.

This principle of providing the indirect service in order to impact the broadest population was evident in the case of the black worker. Even though short-term counseling aimed at providing the worker with a different perspective on the supervisor's comments and developing assertive skills in coping with the supervisor may have reduced the presenting problem, it would have impacted only one individual. Thus, it would not have been as cost effective as a more indirect approach. Instead, when the consultant provides appropriate feedback and support to the supervisor/consultee, the resultant change in the supervisor's behavior may not only impact the individual worker in question, but also may have similar positive effects on all present and future workers under this supervisor's direction.

Consulting Process

Like counseling and other forms of human service practice, consultation can be broken down into a number of stages. Although the stages may be presented as somewhat static, it must be remembered that in practice the process of consultation is active and, therefore, will not occur in a neat, static order, but will move back and forth across the various stages.

Gaining Entry. The first stage of any consult is for the consultant to gain entry into the organization or into the "world" of the consultee. Essential to this process of gaining access is for the consultant to establish the contract for this unique relationship. The consultant should be clear as to the special requirements of the consultation process. The consultant needs to inform the consultee and his/her system that consultation is a collaborative process. Further, the consultee should be helped to understand that the underlying objective of consultation is to impact the largest number of individuals with the least effort through the involvement of all of the significant others in that client's environment.

During the negotiation, the consultant should be clear as to what responsibilities he/she will assume, while at the same time highlighting the reciprocal nature of the consultation relationship.

Problem Identification. Following successful contracting, the consultant must begin to identify the problem at hand. During this stage, the consultant attempts to decide which form of consultation (i.e., direct service to client, indirect service to client) appears most appropriate for this case. Using observational procedures, survey, and structured interviews, the consultant begins to grasp the nature of the problem and the various strategies unsuccessfully tried. While we have attempted to encourage the reader to attempt to consult at the most indirect level of service delivery, it is important to note that in order for the consultant to be effective, he/she must be able to work within the system. Therefore, it is important to work at whatever level one will be allowed—while attempting to move to more indirect forms. Gaining acceptance requires that the consultant be sure to meet the immediate, perceived need of the consultee, in order to demonstrate his/her own usefulness.

Defining the Problem. The third stage is the problem definition stage. During this stage the consultant and consultee develop a detailed definition of the problem. As part of this stage, the consultant has the consultee gather specific data that provide clear, concrete examples of the problem under investigation, along with data that reflect the way the problem is impacted under different environmental conditions. Again, the use of systematic observation is an important means of data collection. Throughout the data collection, the consultant should be encouraging and supportive of the consultee's efforts. In most cases the consultee is unfamiliar with such data collection techniques and may be anxious about his/her level of competence. Providing the consultee with praise and support will go a long way to make for a successful, productive consultation relationship.

Intervening. Following the clear definition of the problem, intervention strategies are developed. At this juncture it is important to highlight the collaborative, educative nature of the consultation relationship. It is essential that the intervention plan that is to be developed reflects the input of the consultee. Unless the consultee feels that it is *his/her* intervention plan, he/she will be less than willing or enthusiastic about implementing the plan.

This point is extremely important since, by definition, a consultation intervention strategy requires the consultee's involvement for implementation. Since the plan is only as good as its implementation, the consultant who collaborates with the consultee and helps him/her feel like an essential contributor to the development of the plan will increase the plan's probability of success.

The specifics of such intervention will obviously vary according to the nature and circumstances of the problem but, in general, often involve providing information either to the client, consultee, or organization; adjusting system or individual policy and procedures; or simply encouraging self-exploration and expression.

Evaluating the Consultation. The fifth stage of consultation involves the assessment of the consultation. Such an evaluation involves gathering data on the impact of the strategy implemented, as well as gathering consultee feedback regarding the nature of the consultation process. All too often this phase is overlooked.

It should be emphasized that this evaluation phase can serve two functions. First, the assessment can be used to demonstrate the consultant's effectiveness and thus provide a basis from which to negotiate the next contract. Secondly, such assessment will provide the feedback needed for the consultant's own professional growth.

Ending the Relationship. The last stage of consultation is concluding or ending the relationship. The effective consultant attempts to place the consultee and/or the organization in such a position that his/her services are no longer needed. This requires that the consultant not only provide competency and training to the consultee, but also foster the consultee's independence. While encouraging self-reliance, the consultant needs to ensure the consultee that he/she will be available should the need arise with this or future problems.

Pitfalls in Consultation

All too often consultation is simplistically equated with sitting, chatting, and drinking coffee. On the contrary, successful consultation is a difficult task. Since the consultant is to function as a facilitator, rather than a director—establishing a fine balance between being viewed as an expert with all of the answers, and being viewed as a colleague with whom one can mutually work and resolve problems—is difficult to manage.

All too often the presence of a consultant signals to the consultee or the system that something is wrong and, thus, needs to be fixed. The idea that something is "wrong" often stimulates anxiety among those who feel they may be accountable. The consultant needs to overcome this perception of the consultant as an "evaluator" or "hatchet person." Without attending to possible sources of resistance and anxiety about the consulting process, the consultant's efforts will more than likely prove quite unproductive. Regardless of the level of consultation, the most carefully conceived recommendations and strategies are doomed to failure if the consultation relationship is less than facilitative because the consultant has failed to minimize the effects of resistance.

Consultation is by definition a process of change, and both systems and individuals tend to resist change. Even though one may agree that a problem exists, one may feel accountable and, thus, act defensively and even attempt to deny responsibility for the situation. Often the consultee will attempt to focus on external factors as causing the problem, rather than accepting the role he/she has played in the creation or maintenance of the problem. A primary goal of consultation is to help such a consultee to accept his/her responsibility for the problem. This acceptance will lead naturally to an acceptance and willingness to participate in the process of problem resolution.

Even when the consultee is willing to accept responsibility for both the problem and problem resolution, resistance may still be experienced. The personal characteristics of the consultant, the philosophical orientation of the consultant, or the atmosphere of the consultation process may be such that it leads to increased anxiety in the consultee and to a desire to avoid and resist the consultant's efforts. A good consultant, like all help-givers, needs to be very sensitive to the nature and quality of the interpersonal relationship involved, and employ those interpersonal skills discussed in part one to facilitate this process.

Summary

The ever increasing demand for human services and the inability to supply the community with adequate numbers of well-trained professionals to meet this demand has led to the development of alternative modes of service delivery. Consultation, as presented within this chapter, is one such service delivery method that over the last ten years has gained in popularity. This increased popularity is in part due to the fact that consultation offers mental health specialists and human service workers a model for impacting the largest number of people possible. Further, the value of consultation appears to lie in acting not only as a method of providing remediation, but also as a method of preventive mental health services.

Consultation has all too often been simplistically associated with the process of "advice giving" or "chatting." As outlined within the chapter, consultation is instead a very complicated, interpersonal process that demands great sophistication and planning. The successful consultant needs to be able to enter into a system or organization exhibiting a problem; to identify and define the problem; to work *in collaboration* with the consultee; to develop intervention strategies that are evaluated for their effectiveness; and finally to terminate the relationship. This entire process demands that the consultant not only be skilled in appropriate diagnostic and remedial strategies, but also in those interpersonal skills necessary for the creation of a facilitative, collaborative relationship.

12 / allied health professionals

Up to this point, we have concerned ourselves with those areas clearly within the scope of helping people. However, skills in gathering information (i.e., diagnosis), as well as providing direct care (i.e., counseling) and indirect consultative services are not the only ones necessary when working with people.

Today, the allied health professional will be called upon to serve in a variety of roles—as team member, supervisor, educator, and community mental health facilitator. Each role is vital to the problems of the modern health movement and each role brings with it special demands.

Team Member

First and foremost, allied health professionals are part of a team. Whether they serve as counselors in a community mental health center, as physician's assistants in a group practice, as assistant caseworkers, or as licensed practical nurses in a hospital setting, allied health professionals must function as team members. Being an integral part of the treatment group has implications in terms of added responsibilities and problems that differ from those associated with working alone with individual patients. For example, as a team member the health professional must be able to communicate effectively with superiors co-workers, and subordinates.

Superiors. Dealing with one's direct supervisor or superior can be quite difficult for personnel in newly established positions. People in the traditional professions of social work, medicine, and psychology—such as caseworkers, internists, psychologists, and psychiatrists—are inclined to show some resentment toward such titles as physician's assistant, counselor's aid, assistant caseworker, and mental health worker. They may see the development of these positions as threats to their own status or employment stability, or may even oppose the use of associate professionals on philosophical grounds. Overcoming such negative attitudes can be accomplished by demonstrating a willingness to learn and perform in a satisfactory manner, so as to supplement and lend support to the roles of those in traditional positions. Hostility should not be taken personally, but rather understood as a transitory prejudice toward change that will diminish and eventually disappear as the new positions become routine.

On the brighter side, the number of settings in which allied health professionals are welcome as team members is on the increase, and there is already some lessening of friction and suspicion among those in traditional treatment roles. With this acceptance, frank communication with superiors develops naturally and easily.

Co-workers. While keeping one's supervisors informed is important, they are not the only ones with whom the allied health professional must communicate. Co-workers must also be kept abreast of one's professional activities in the center, hospital, clinic, or particular job setting in which the team operates. Since co-workers may come from different backgrounds and have varied kinds of training, this should be kept in mind when they are briefed in small groups, so that information concerning, for example, a client or treatment management situation will be communicated with minimal distortions. A few simple rules can be helpful:

1. Involve each individual in the dialogue to avoid the appearance of talking down or discouraging participation. (This is important to remember when conducting ward rounds or when in a conference with others from different disciplines who might find your profession's technical language or jargon unfamiliar.)
2. Develop the material slowly and logically. Avoid jumping from topic to topic or conveying a great deal of information too quickly.
3. In addition to responding to actual questions, encourage comments or queries from those whose facial expressions show puzzlement or surprise.

With experience, workers tend to develop effective personal techniques to facilitate communication and to avoid harmful misunderstandings. Communication with co-workers is a process requiring constant attention.

Subordinates. Gaining acceptance when entering a new organization can be a painful experience for the worker. Newly appointed supervisors occasionally aggravate the uneasiness of workers by their failure to keep lines of communication open, often because they have simply forgotten their own frustrations and problems when they occupied subordinate positions.

The following list suggests several ways communication may be interrupted or distorted by supervisors who fail to remain alert to their subordinates' problems.

1. Providing solutions in lieu of providing ample opportunity for problem-solving efforts.
2. Discouraging, rather than facilitating, the amplification of ideas by quickly blaming or offhandedly praising subordinates before they have had the chance to express themselves fully on the matter.
3. Ignoring or humoring the person.
4. Abruptly changing the topic after a subordinate has introduced it.
5. Threatening or insulting an individual as a means of forcing him or her to act in a particular way, without concern for the person's feelings.
6. Being pedantic and ordering others to do something before eliciting any input they might have.

Assistants' comments, questions, and problem-solving efforts should be encouraged. Just as the allied health professional desires acceptance as part of a team, participation in the group decision-making process, and respect as an essential worker, so also does the worker's assistant expect acceptance and respect. Proper regard for the duties and responsibilities of all concerned is essential to the success of the team.

Areas of special concern to the unit director or supervisor are organizational opportunities for self-advancement and professional growth, the need for continuing education, and the importance of performing ethically when serving as a health worker. One of the most sensitive ethical issues concerns the question of confidentiality.

Awareness of the critical importance of confidentiality is something the new worker must acquire and respect. Supervisors should take great care to inform new workers that all information concerning clients is to be kept in the strictest confidence. Such information may be shared only with other treatment personnel; and even when sharing serves the purpose of educating others not involved in the case, the identity of the client is guarded. Circumspection extends to phone conversations when the identity of the caller is uncertain, and the consent of the client is required before information may be given to anyone other than the members of the treatment unit involved.

Supervisor

Supervision presents an opportunity for professional growth. Free discussion of questions, actions, and the difficulties encountered on the job will help to correct mistakes and develop strategies for dealing with future professional challenges. On the other hand, withholding details of how various situations were handled tends to reduce or exclude the benefits that may derive from supervisory responsibility.

It is only natural to wish to appear in full control of any situation and to attempt to interpret what happened in order to avoid being seen in an unfavorable light. Repression is a sign of this problem, as when it seems difficult to remember what occurred during a counseling session. This may result from unconscious attempts to block out or repress failures or mistakes made with a client during a session, and serves to keep potentially damaging information from the supervisor. Rationalizing when reporting to a supervisor can best be countered by taking time to recall details of what occurred during a session, and this should be done as soon as possible after the session has ended. Rather than offering interpretations of what happened by means of phrases such as, "The patient seemed to be angry," the counselor should repeat the client's verbal reactions, together with his own responses.

> "The client frowned and said, 'I think you're keeping information from me.' "
> "I responded, 'Why do you say that?' but I felt queasy in my stomach since I thought she was putting me on the spot."

Recalling the precise details of a session requires effort, but usually brings valuable feedback from an experienced supervisor. The supervisor should therefore be seen as a concerned helper whose assistance is vital to successful therapy.

Since most people are sensitive to criticism, a supervisor's comments should be presented with a good deal of tact. Callously pointing to mistakes can have the negative effect of causing the worker to fear candor and to resist suggestions for change or improvement.

The successful supervisor will also take care to allow workers sufficient time to explain their actions and to discuss alternative ways of approaching particular situations. If a supervisor believes the worker has made a poor choice in his or her method of dealing with a client, an alternative should be suggested as gently as possible.

Here is a brief list of suggestions to be followed when eliciting information.

1. Try to put the worker at ease through a brief introductory conversation about some common topic of interest or through light humor.
2. Allow the worker to review the session in detail.
3. Upon completion of a report of either part or all of the session, elicit any questions the worker might have.
4. Encourage the worker to answer without fear of being prematurely cut off, having the end point of his or her comment or question anticipated, or being harshly criticized even on minor points.

5. Provide positive comments instead of interrupting the worker with ways in which the situation could have been handled more effectively.

The supervisor is first and foremost a consultant, rather than a commander who orders or demands. The supervisor is not the worker's therapist, a common error of novice supervisors.

Personality conflicts are bound to occur from time to time, and in such an instance the conflict should be recognized and briefly discussed. Extensive analysis should not be undertaken by those involved; this is a matter for another therapist.

Persuading an individual to change his or her style of dealing with others is difficult for a variety of reasons. To some, this change means that to a certain degree they must lose face and admit that past, personal techniques were wrong and that they as individuals are ineffectual. This admission also makes them dependent on someone else for guidance in how to apply new, possibly strange, styles that may be difficult to learn and may lead to criticism when they are not applied properly. As a result, some workers will resist learning and changing by using many types of ploys. To deal effectively with these tactics, the supervisor should attempt to phrase corrections in the least threatening manner possible.

"All right, let's see, you handled _____ by doing _____. Let's stop and see what other ways you might have handled it." (Time given for person to come up with and go over alternatives.)

"Aha, good. One other way I suggest you consider is _____. The reason I mention this approach is _____."

The supervisor also needs to be aware of some of the tactics workers might employ to avoid discussing the techniques they use when conducting a counseling session. Such tactics might include changing the topic, praising the supervisor, speaking at length about the worker's personal life, talking about nonprofessional topics or questions of a professional nature that are unrelated to the present discussion.

The supervisor should be prepared to deal with these and similar ploys. This can be done by moving the session back onto the topic. For example, if a worker starts asking professional questions that are unrelated to the topic, the supervisor might say, "Maybe we can chat about _____ later. Why don't we speak for awhile about the counseling session you just had with Mr. _____ because one of the interesting patterns Mr. _____ is demonstrating is _____."

Educator

Many allied health professionals are educators, as well as supervisors. In this capacity, they are often called upon to give brief lectures to groups in preservice and inservice training programs.

An individual who is given the task of teaching a class for the first time will naturally be anxious. Yet, by following a number of simple rules, the lecture can be designed to provide the maximum amount of pertinent data in the time allotted.

Rule 1: Be familiar with the material to be covered. Facing an audience ill prepared can be a devastating experience for both the lecturer and the listeners. Having an idea of what one wants to cover is not sufficient. The instructor must actually be prepared.

Rule 2: Know the key issues and problems. Every subject area includes topics that deserve more attention than others because of their importance, complexity, or uniqueness. Likewise, most subjects have certain problem areas that need special coverage in order to help the student or novice trainee deal with them effectively.

Rule 3: Make the issues involved alive and relevant. If the audience does not see the relevance or practicability of the information given, they will dismiss or screen out much of it long before they have had a chance to examine it in even a perfunctory way. Consequently, whenever possible, the lecturer should use illustrations and examples to show the relevance of the information being disseminated. For instance, if an individual is giving a lecture on interviewing techniques to practical nurse trainees, he or she will want to use illustrations of how nursing personnel can employ the inter-personal techniques being provided.

Rule 4: Encourage participation. One point that should be stressed from the onset of the lecture is that the only poor question is the one left unasked. If time and material permit, the lecturer should encourage class partici-pation. This can be accomplished during the lecture by asking the students open-ended discussion questions. This will not only increase attention, but in many instances will also enhance a better, more sophisticated apprecia-tion of the material.

Ideally, when possible, breaking down the group into small subgroups after a short lecture is a good learning technique. In small group students can discuss their opinions, questions, and recommendations on the area in question. One of the students can act as recorder and present a synthesis of what was said to the whole class at the end of the instructional period. If staffing permits, another approach would be to include in each group an allied health professional experienced in the area under discussion, so he or she can serve as group leader. Whatever the approach, it is beneficial if time can be set aside for structured group discussion of the material being presented.

Rule 5: Summarize material. At the end of even a brief session, key points of the lecture should be reemphasized. Such a review reinforces the knowledge already gained from the lecture, by putting it in overall per-spective. This is done through the use of an end-of-class summary.

Community Mental Health Facilitator

Whether promoting the client's welfare in a hospital, residential unit, or community clinic or center, allied health professionals need to be aware of other resources that are available to the client. While it is true that the client often has personal talents that are untapped and that the hospital or clinic has facilities the client should be encouraged to utilize, it is also necessary for the staff to involve the client's family in the treatment. Thus it is equally important to help the client become aware of what the open community has to offer.

Family. In the past, traditional therapies concentrated on the individual and neglected the client's family. Today, mental health treatment personnel are beginning to appreciate the impact the family has on the client's well-being—whether by maintaining or exacerbating the client's problems, or by providing positive support.

Interpersonal conflicts between family members—particularly between the client and his or her spouse or parents—can be examined when families are brought in for treatment. Even if the family is brought in for just one or several short consultation sessions, these can still prove useful, for under such circumstances family members may begin to become involved in the therapeutic work needed to alleviate the client's current problems.

People cannot be separated from their environments. For example, it is senseless to help a person to handle a gastrointestinal problem by informing him what medicine he should take and what foods he should avoid if his wife insists on feeding him food that is contraindicated for his condition. As noted in chapter 5, the system in which the client lives and to which he or she will return must also be analyzed and treated if the client's treatment is to be effective. This type of involvement is particularly necessary in short-term counseling.

The Community. The community is also in a position to offer various specialized supportive assistance. Accordingly, allied health professionals should be aware of the types of community services which are available to the patient (see table 12.1).

By knowing what community resources, particularly local ones (i.e., in the neighborhood and within walking distance), are available, the worker can often involve the community in the *initial* planning phase of the treatment. This can be useful, for if an outside resource sees that it is being involved from the beginning, it may be more apt to cooperate than if called upon as an afterthought.

The allied health professional must resist playing the role of "the one and only helper." All too often one can start to believe that no one else

Table 12.1. Community Services: A Partial List of Categories

Mental Health
    Psychiatric outpatient clinics
    Crisis units—residential and nonresidential
    Hotlines (suicide, drugs, AA)
    Community mental health centers
    Mental retardation services
Family
    Family planning
    Marital counseling
    Adoption–foster care services
Senior Citizens
    Nursing homes
    Senior citizen clubs
Criminal Justice
    Police
    Courts
    Corrections (institutions, community-based centers)
    Probation and parole
    Legal aid
Drugs
    AA
    Halfway houses
Education
    Preschool
    Daycare
    High school equivalency programs
    Adult education
    Evening classes
    GI Bill
Employment
    Government
    Private
    Resume services
Medical
    Clinics
    Special care facilities or services (blind, deaf, diabetic, venereal disease...)
    Visiting nurses
Social Services
    Welfare
    Private social services agencies
Vocational/Occupational
    VA
    Sheltered workshops
    State employment agencies
Miscellaneous
    Aliens
    Church services
    Housing services (YMCA, Boarding houses, group homes)

could do as much for the client or really care as much as oneself. Such an orientation is not only inaccurate, but if maintained will surely add to the worker's already overwhelming case load and surely increase the possibility of worker burnout.

The worker needs to recognize that regardless of the wealth or apparent poverty of a community, other people, groups, agencies, etc., exist and are concerned about the client and his/her problems. Learning how to join with them and function as a team, in a cooperative, collaborative effort, should be our aim. It is through such a cooperative effort that we can truly maximize the depth and breadth of our helping efforts.

Cultural Issues. Probably one of the main reasons allied health professionals should involve the community in the treatment from the start is that there are cultural differences between them and much of their treatment population. No matter how sophisticated the worker's training is, there are barriers between the client and the treatment agent that cannot be quickly broken down.

This should not be surprising. For example, if the worker is a Caucasian from suburbia and the client is a black or Chicano who has always lived in an urban ghetto, the client may feel negatively toward the worker because of previous unpleasant associations with Caucasians (e.g., police, social worker, absentee landlord). In addition, it is natural for some members of certain minority groups to resent help from an outsider. Since it is through solidarity with other members of their social, racial, or neighborhood group that they manage to develop and preserve enough pride and identity to ward off despair, fragmentation, and failure, this should not be surprising.

Even in cases in which the client who comes from a different background from the treatment agent is willing to accept treatment, the treatment may not fulfill the client's needs because the agent may be unaware of certain needs this person has because of his or her different life style or unique environmental situation. While the allied health professional may be concerned with the client's personality, he or she may ignore or minimize more basic needs, such as housing and finances. A community worker who is aware that basic survival is an issue in the case would not make the same mistake. Therefore, allied health professional should begin to look upon community personnel as essential, rather than second-class assistants—a view held by too many allied and traditional health professionals.

If we are to become involved in and deal effectively with the overwhelming problems of our cities, we must be willing to credit the community with the ability to help instead of to hinder the client's efforts to get better. Just as the allied health movement is a testament to shared power in the treatment professions today, efforts to involve the open community in working with people is a logical extension of the tenet that helping the emotionally and physically incapacitated is the concern of *all* people, not just a select few.

Summary

The role of the allied health professional is often multifacted and quite varied. This chapter attempted to delineate the special role demands faced by the professional who is in a position of mental health team member, supervisor educator, or community facilitator.

Each of the roles discussed requires the mental health professional to possess specialized talents and skills. As a team member, the worker needs to apply group principles in facilitating a collabortive environment. Keeping channels of communication open to co-workers and superiors is essential to team functioning. Further, as a supervisor, the mental health worker needs to be able to provide feedback clearly and constructively to others seeking professional growth. Observational skills and the ability to provide feedback are essential to the role of supervisor. Finally, the chapter presented a number of specific considerations for the creation, organization, and implementation of educational and community based programs.

appendixes

a / counseling keystones

This section consists of a brief collection of statements on the theory and practice of counseling.* The statements are provided to encourage reflection on the relevance and applicability of certain counseling principles and techniques.

The section is arranged so that several statements are on each page. All on them are categorized under four headings:

1. Keystones related to the counselor.
2. Keystones related to the client.
3. Keystones related to the counseling relationship.
4. Keystones related to counseling skills, techniques, and goals.

The reader's pace will no doubt vary depending upon his or her immediate needs and interests, and how these are touched upon by any one or group of statements.

It is hoped that, in thinking about the statements, the reader will be able to gain a better insight into how she or he does, or might, interact with a counseling client. Though this section can be skimmed through quickly, it is hoped that because of the stated purpose of increasing self-awareness in the counseling process, the reader will pace him- or herself in order to get the most out of the counseling keystones.

Keystones Related to the Counselor

No matter how forceful, active, or directive a counselor feels she must be during a session, she normally should not relieve the client of the responsibility to act in his own behalf.

*   *   *

Though a counselor naturally should not promise the client a miracle, she can still offer him some hope that alleviation of the symptoms of his problems can be expected.

*   *   *

---

* In this appendix feminine pronouns will be used to designate the counselor and male pronouns, to refer to the client.

If a counselor can link a client's distressing complaints to some of his more basic problems, the client might be more apt to consider the complaints as important rather than as unimportant and worthy of dismissal.

* * *

If the client feels the counselor is pressing him, he may act or speak in a surprisingly unreasonable fashion. The counselor must consider this possibility when deciding upon the pace of the session, or she will be caught off guard by the client's hostile or unusually emotional reaction.

* * *

Counseling is set back or ceases the instant a counselor reacts emotionally in terms of her own needs rather than those of the client.

* * *

The counselor does not usually intervene directly to physically eliminate or correct a problem. What she does is act to change the client's outlook so he can deal with it himself.

* * *

No matter how nondirective or superficial the counseling may be, if the counselor is unaware of the assets and liabilities of her own personality, she will usually be ineffective and sometimes cause great harm.

* * *

If the counselor believes she should interpret the client's behavior for him, she should give the explanation in logical, structured, and understandable terms, rather than in psychological jargon.

* * *

If the counselor wants to make an important point, she should repeat it in different ways to the client at various counseling junctures to see that it is firmly impressed in his mind.

* * *

A counselor may gain insight into a new client's behavior response patterns by giving him hypothetical situations and having him think and fantasize out loud about his reactions to them.

* * *

A sense of humor is a trait that the counselor should not suppress, but use in counseling to help the client become relaxed and flexible enough to enjoy the incongruities in his environment and the foolish aspects of his behavior.

* * *

In summarizing and clarifying the client's behavior, the counselor should use comparisons. By comparing two issues, feelings, actions, or thoughts expressed by the client, the client should find it easy to see contradictions and patterns in them.

*   *   *

The counselor has little or no knowledge of a new client's real feelings, beliefs, and ideas. Therefore, in the early phases of counseling even an apparently weak agreement with what he says about himself can be a mistake.

*   *   *

The disparity between the client's purported and real goals must be recognized and thoroughly understood by the counselor so that she can indirectly bring this information to the client's attention at the proper time.

*   *   *

"Am I clear about the reason that I am effective or a failure with certain clients and problems." This question is one a counselor must continually ask herself.

*   *   *

In summarizing the session, the counselor has an opportunity to emphasize certain aspects of the client's comments and projected feelings. This process enables the client to readily see the importance of some of his statements, a realization that otherwise might have been lost among the other less essential things said during the session.

*   *   *

Labeling clients ("neurotic," "inadequate")—especially early in counseling—can be misleading. Instead, the counselor might note her initial impressions of the client by picturing him on a series of scales such as self-image, dependency-independency, impulsivity, maturity, sociability.

*   *   *

Reasoning with a person about changing his unusual or self-defeating behavior is not the job of the counselor. She appreciates that the client's emotionally toned attitudes will not be altered simply by providing a strong rational argument.

*   *   *

When a client asks why he is having a problem, the counselor should take this opportunity to explore with him the secondary gains he is receiving for acting inappropriately.

*   *   *

If a person casually reveals a feeling, idea, or belief that the counselor feels is of particular importance, she should have the client repeat it in order to make him aware of its value.

*   *   *

While values are not imposed by a counselor, the implications of a client's code of living are still open to examination since they will have an impact on the client's search for personal fulfillment.

*   *   *

A secure counselor does not become defensive when a client opposes or attacks her on an issue or on the usefulness of a counseling technique.

* * *

A counseling technique that fails may be an indication that the counselor's appraisal of the person or his problem is inaccurate.

* * *

Unless the counselor periodically interrupts the counseling process to clarify the client's statements and feelings, she will be unable to determine if her impressions are acceptable to the client.

* * *

Even if the counselor does not believe the client's real problem is the one that initially caused him to ask for help, the client's reported problem should still be considered during treatment.

* * *

Counseling is an active, malleable process. At one point a client may be providing unimportant data; at the next he could be revealing relevant information. One of the roles of the counselor is to connect and emphasize the essential, meaningful aspects of the session, so that they are not clouded by the less important factors.

* * *

Feedback is not advice. The information a counselor gives to a client is meant to help him make his own decision.

* * *

In a conversation or discussion, people often measure their involvement by the amount they say. In counseling (a purposeful conversation) the counselor's involvement is not measured in this manner, for she is more often operating as an active listener.

* * *

Being tactful and respectful of a client's feelings does not mean that the counselor should present diluted truths or ignore important points because they are unpleasant. It merely means that care should be taken not to be unnecessarily direct or brutal in bringing up or discussing issues.

* * *

Every counselor makes mistakes, distorts reality, and develops some form of countertransference (unrealistic attitudes toward the client). However, the adept counselor eventually recognizes and admits her errors, so she can calibrate for them when dealing with the client.

* * *

When the counselor imposes time limits, she is merely confronting the client with a reality: namely, the counselor has only so much time to spend with each client.

Accordingly, it is *up to the client* to make the most of the time allotment.

* * *

All of the decisions made by the client during counseling will not lead to action. One of the counselor's jobs is to distinguish between the decisions the client makes that will lead to action and those that are not going to result in change.

* * *

The counselor's acceptance of the client—with all of his problems and personal liabilities—helps the client to accept himself.

* * *

When the counselor uses nondogmatic phrases ("I feel . . .," "It seems to me . . ."), she is less likely to evoke defensiveness on the part of the client.

* * *

Prior to initiation of the process of clarification, the counselor must reflect on the specific areas she wants to cover and the points she plans to emphasize.

* * *

A good counselor gives the client the impression that she is sharing information with him, not just talking to him.

* * *

When the client has problems, the counselor must not only seek to find out *why*, trying to make, but instead attempt to keep as open a mind as possible.

* * *

In clarifying what the client has said, the counselor must be careful not to put words in his mouth.

* * *

When the client has problems, the counselor must not only seek to find out *why*, she also needs to determine *when* and *with whom* he is having difficulties.

* * *

Prior to questioning and commenting, the counselor should be aware of how she plans to phrase the information she will try to communicate. In addition, she should be alert to the potential reactions she can expect from the client.

* * *

In summarizing the content of the session, the counselor is expected not only to synthesize the factual content, but also the feelings that the client attaches to each issue.

* * *

Every person is continuously caught between two opposing views when he is called upon to make a decision on day-to-day issues. Yet, such daily conflicts can be resolved by the person who is able to approach the problem logically. Such training in resolving daily conflicts is offered to people who enter counseling, if the counselor is aware of her total role.

* * *

The client's goals for entering counseling are important. Though this principle should seem quite evident, too often the counselor develops her own set of goals for the client to the point that the client's expressed aims are lost.

* * *

Lack of interest in the client is occasionally excused (rationalized) by the counselor on the grounds that close involvement with him would reduce her ability to be objective.

* * *

While observing the client, the counselor must also remember to monitor her own feelings, comments, and reactions; this is often forgotten by the counseling student after she has had some minimal experience.

* * *

Unless a counselor is able to help a client to deal with his immediate, living world, her work will be ineffective.

* * *

Naturally, the client should be called upon to describe how he believes he is different from other people. However, he should also be further prompted to describe the variances *within his own* behavior pattern. Thus, the counselor should explore with the client why he thinks or acts in one way at a particular time and in a different way at other times.

* * *

By being patient, the counselor teaches the client to be patient.

* * *

When a counselor is silent during the session, she should be listening, not just waiting for an opportunity to talk.

* * *

Being able to remember the "little things" the client says can be one of the biggest assets a counselor can possess.

* * *

Acceptance does not mean that the counselor ignores or denies a client's deficiencies. It means instead that she does not reject the client on the basis of these limitations.

* * *

Words of approval or support cease to have an impact if they are used too often by the counselor.

*   *   *

When a client relates a story, he usually gives only his version of the events. He does not tell how other people might have perceived the interaction. The counselor must allow for this when she listens to the client.

*   *   *

Manifest content (what is said) never totally equals the full content (the *complete* meaning) of the statement made by a client. Unless the counselor is alert, she will risk making the mistake of accepting what the client says at face value.

*   *   *

If the counselor is adept enough to get the client to realistically recreate an important scene in his life, she will be able to better visualize the event. Moreover, such a dramatization, in itself, will be beneficial for the client.

*   *   *

A good listener does not speak too often. Since a counselor must learn to listen *actively*, her experience and comfortableness in the session can often be measured by how often she speaks.

*   *   *

Before asking the client a question, the counselor should prepare herself for the client's reaction by considering the possible responses that he might give.

*   *   *

A counselor does not provide answers. Rather, she helps the client to ultimately arrive at his own conclusions.

*   *   *

A counselor's anxiety during the counseling session should not be ignored or suppressed. Unless it is faced and dealt with, the counselor will never grow professionally.

*   *   *

In being concerned about the client's liabilities, the counselor must not forget to recognize his assets as well.

*   *   *

Referral or background information on a client is a collection of information that has been selected by a person or persons. Since such a selection implies that certain data have been excluded, the counselor must always assume that the information she gets is incomplete.

*   *   *

If a counselor is not constantly alert, she may subtly influence a client to take a particular course of action that may not be in accord with his philosophy of life.

* * *

A counselor gives a client's life meaning when she helps him to realize that he is a person with the potential to make living rewarding.

* * *

The client may only be capable of illogical self-analysis when he enters counseling. The counselor's role then is to aid him in beginning logical self-exploration and in learning to appreciate why he was unable to accomplish such a self-examination in the past. This is important in preventing similar difficulties when counseling is terminated and the client is on his own again.

* * *

In serving as a guide, the counselor is concerned with pointing out the pivotal issues complicating the major problems a client has.

* * *

A person may feel that the only way to self-understanding is to look into himself. In counseling, the counselor should also make the client aware that he can get a good image of himself by pondering the types of friends he has, his interests and values, and the daily pursuits he finds rewarding.

* * *

Though there may seem to be a great distance between the counselor and the client during his first several sessions with her, she should not be discouraged, because at that point she may be closer to him than anyone else.

Keystones Related to the Client

With the counselor's support, the client should be able to challenge some of his own basic assumptions concerning life, reality, and interpersonal relations.

* * *

Once a person sees that his method of adapting to life is not the only one open to him, he can begin to explore alternative forms of goal-seeking and problem-solving behavior.

* * *

Many clients have relinquished conscious control over their lives. They have lost the desire or strength to challenge the primary philosophy that now dominates their existence.

* * *

When a client has the opportunity to communicate his vague feelings and problems by *reducing* them to specific words and patterns, he often begins to feel some control over them again.

* * *

A person who says he has difficulty controlling his aggressive impulses is also saying that he is afraid to face and deal with his insecurities.

* * *

The opinions an individual forms of people and things are always changing. As he grows and moves through developmental stages, it is natural that his views (including his opinions of the people close to him) become altered. If an individual fails to realize this, he will usually feel a great deal of guilt.

* * *

As soon as the client realizes that his problem is not unique and that the counselor accepts him despite his claimed weakness or inadequacies, his sense of hopelessness will begin to diminish.

* * *

Self-confidence in the client will increase if in his daily life he is able to successfully link his distressing feelings with their causes.

* * *

A client must learn to be his own detective. When he has mood swings, he should become accustomed to asking himself, "Why do I feel this way?" and "Who and what makes me react in this manner?"

* * *

Most clients' problems are partially related to their solutions. (For example, a marginal student would rather study the subjects he likes than the one he's failing; a shy bachelor only dates women he's sure will accept his invitation to go out with him.)

* * *

The client should occasionally be called upon to present his view of what the role of the counselor should be in order to see how his perceptions in this area are developing.

* * *

A desirable anticipated result—no matter how improbable—is one of the most motivating forces a person can have to continue acting in an unreasonable fashion (e.g., a spurned lover who continues to follow and keep in touch with his former girlfriend in the hopes that she will *eventually* return to him).

* * *

How does the client believe the significant persons in his life view him? This is a question that the client should be asked to answer.

*   *   *

While a client vaguely knows that he needs help, he may still openly deny this fact even though he has actively sought out a counselor. Such resistance is natural and should lessen as counseling proceeds and a relationship is formed.

*   *   *

Just as the client's efforts and positive thinking should be supported, his inappropriate actions and the problems that result from them should not be rewarded with sympathy.

*   *   *

A client will become more independent as soon as he begins to realize that his life's direction is affected by his own skills and attitudes.

*   *   *

Pressing the client to discuss meaningful material early in the counseling session accomplishes little. He must be allowed to present fairly neutral material until he is able to form a relationship with the counselor.

*   *   *

Many clients are frustrated because of the unattainable goals they set for themselves. These goals are often based on irrational, simplistic views: (1) if a person acts properly, everyone will like him; and (2) either a person is totally competent or he is completely inadequate.

*   *   *

The client must learn to postulate new potential areas of interest for himself without losing the organizational ability to see which of them is ultimately unrealistic.

*   *   *

A client's choice can be termed "good" if it helps him to improve his relationship with others without diminishing his own self-image.

*   *   *

A breakthrough is achieved in the counseling of a new client when he shares a problem that makes him feel guilty or embarrassed.

*   *   *

To succeed in counseling, a client may not have to replace the tenets he has lived by; rather, he may only be required to put things in their proper perspective.

*   *   *

The more a person is able to see how (and, if possible, from whom) he acquired information that led to the formation of the opinions he now has, the less sacred they will be; as a result, he will become more willing to consider changing them.

*   *   *

Though the counseling session is limited by the time, the client's self-actualizing process is not. Even when the actual meeting with the counselor is over, the opportunity for the client to grow continues.

* * *

When a client begins to enjoy being himself, counseling has made an impact.

* * *

Rejection of, or resistance to, the information the counselor provides can be caused by a client's misinterpretation of what the counseling objectives should be. Such problems usually diminish as soon as the client becomes familiar with the counselor's style, and flexible enough to lower his defenses and examine the incoming data.

* * *

Until a client can communicate a plan of action in *specific* terms, he is not ready to implement it.

* * *

One problem that often appears in counseling is that the client views his difficulties in either too limited or global a manner.

* * *

A person will become more responsive to counseling when he begins to realize that self-examination not only leads to a discovery of his limitations, but also to an uncovering of his potential, in the form of untapped personal resources.

* * *

In counseling, the person should begin to see how much effort he exerts to please others at the expense of his own happiness.

* * *

The fact that a client firmly defends a life style that he knows is unworkable is proof that he is in need of great assistance and support.

* * *

When a client is examining his behavior, he usually tries to report why he believes he did something. However, the counselor should also elicit from him how he felt immediately prior to, and following, the act.

* * *

Truth is unattainable for the client who is not ready for self-revelation.

* * *

When a person uses superlatives (i.e., "never," "always"), the counselor must view the statements in which they were employed with a degree of skepticism.

* * *

When relating a concept, a client should be required to tie it to events and circumstances in his life. As a result, his comments will become more meaningful.

* * *

Just as a person is often responsible for limiting himself, he also has the power to realize his potential.

* * *

When a client is called on continually to describe his perceptions and compare them with the views of other people, his understanding of reality usually improves.

* * *

If a client can measure his improvement by concrete elements in his life (e.g., weight loss, increased participation in creative pursuits), he may be more apt to accept the counselor's statement that he is growing in areas that are less definiable (self-respect).

* * *

The counselor must aid the client who does not know what he wants in life to develop general goals and to tailor these broad objectives to his particular life style.

* * *

A client may share his feelings and perceptions to see if they are accurate and also to find out if others have them as well.

* * *

The people who originally seem to be the most motivated to seek counseling are often the ones most hesitant to become involved in a meaningful interpersonal relationship with the counselor.

* * *

Growth in counseling accelerates for the client when he begins to accept the fact that positive self-control and self-direction may sometimes be painful to effect.

* * *

When the client sees that the counselor accepts him as an individual, he must learn that this means he should also respect other people's rights to act and believe according to their own philosophies.

* * *

Anxiety may be caused by a person's inaccurate perception of a situation rather than by the actual presence of a problem.

* * *

Before beginning counseling, the client usually has done some type of self-analysis. This point should be mentioned to the new client to see what process of self-examination he has gone through and what he believes he has accomplished in the way of self-knowledge.

* * *

A client is often upset and confused when he comes to a counselor not only because he is faced with many conflicting self-values and problems, but also because of the pain, vague fear, and frustration he has experienced in trying to solve them.

* * *

Rational information is often (consciously or unconsciously) dismissed by the emotional client. As a result, knowing what level the client is *primarily* operating on—rational or emotional—at any given time is important.

* * *

One of the questions that the client should be prompted to answer for himself is, "What will happen if I continue to operate within my present life style?"

* * *

In some cases, adjustment for the client may primarily involve his willingness to change his physical environment.

* * *

In the early stages of counseling, it is natural for the client to be confused and concerned about the intentions, responsibilities, and commitment of the counselor.

* * *

For a client, knowing more about his capabilities and interests is not enough. He should also become aware of his current motivations and ultimate goals, or he will find it difficult to plan and implement a personally satisfying style of living.

* * *

Even minimal environmental change initiated by the client usually hurts. He fears the new and is anxious about rejecting the old. Yet he can still venture to take small courageous steps if he feels the support of his counselor.

* * *

When a client points out a trait he likes in the counselor, he is sometimes indirectly saying that this is a characteristic he wishes he had. Likewise, in criticizing the counselor he is often revealing (projecting) some of his own unwanted liabilities.

* * *

Movement in counseling accelerates as soon as: (1) the client understands how he and the counselor can work on his problem in an organized way; (2) he is able to see some of the specific difficulties with which they must deal; and (3) he is sufficiently strong to be willing to take some initial steps.

Keystones Related to the Counseling Relationship

In weaning a client from counseling, the counselor should be fully aware of the type of client with whom she is dealing. In one instance, the dependency relationship with the counselor may be literally keeping the person intact at the time (schizophrenic); in other instances, such as with neurotics, a dependency relationship may prevent clients from growing and maturing.

* * *

A person whose normal sense of mastery is suddenly shattered by the acute onset of a problem may be especially dependent upon the counselor in the first several sessions.

* * *

The dramatic evolution of independence, personality force, and creative positive attitudes is possible when a warm, accepting counseling milieu is experienced by a stifled, sheltered client.

* * *

To establish good rapport with a client, the counselor must be able to indicate to him that she respects the severity of his most pressing problem. This is particularly important because, prior to entering counseling, the client usually finds it difficult to get a noncounselor to appreciate his problem.

* * *

An interpersonal process without emotional content is not counseling. Intellectualizing with the client may be fun, but it will be unproductive in the long run.

* * *

The counselor works with the client to help him identify his current and potential talents. This process is followed by a phase in which the client is given an opportunity to develop these recently discovered assets.

* * *

Building a trust relationship takes time. Often the reason a client does not relate enough information about his true feelings is that he lacks complete trust in the counselor. The counselor should recognize this and have patience; furthermore, she should be careful not to react negatively to the client who is slow in forming a good relationship with her.

* * *

With the counselor's support, the client should become willing to take new steps and alter behavioral patterns, no matter how unusual or futile they might seem.

* * *

If the counselor can get a new client to list what he hates and loves, she may be able to get a quick, unique insight into the person early in the counseling relationship.

* * *

Even in the case of very dependent clients or ones who expect the counselor to have the "answers" to their problems, the counselor must design the counseling situation so the client is prompted to involve himself early in some type of activity that will help correct his difficulties.

*   *   *

During the counseling session, as in any lengthy interpersonal encounter, the attitudes and feelings of the participants will change many times before it is over.

*   *   *

The flow of communication is constricted when the client or counselor becomes anxious or angry. (Anger is often used to veil anxiety.)

*   *   *

The counselor does not have to explain her counseling style to the client. The client will be able to determine a role for himself in relation to the counselor based on his observation of the interpersonal process that evolves during the first several sessions.

*   *   *

The counseling environment must be accepting and warm enough to permit the client to be completely frank about an issue or problem. If the client is convinced that the counselor is able to appreciate his feelings and the environmental pressures that caused him to take certain actions, he will more readily accept the counselor's reactions and comments.

*   *   *

In the counseling setting, the client's anxiety and uncertainty is matched by the counselor's composure and self-confidence.

*   *   *

Individual counseling sessions should be the ideal proving ground for interpersonal development. The atmosphere set up by the counselor should encourage the client to form other relationships, rather than to retreat into a private relationship with the counselor.

*   *   *

A genuine counseling relationship does not arise out of the use of a certain technique, but can only develop when the counselor is willing to invest herself in the process as a *total* person.

*   *   *

When a person enters counseling, he often anticipates either a miracle or a complete failure. One of the steps a counselor should take to deal with this is to indicate in an early session that counseling is not a mysterious, magical event, but a carefully developed series of interpersonal encounters that can aid the client to tap his potential.

*   *   *

When a client enters counseling, he often assumes a dependent position because of the presence of his problem and his prior notions of the role of the counselor. Though such an initial arrangement is natural, the counselor would be wrong to encourage the continuation of such a relationship.

* * *

Age, sex, level of maturity, socioeconomic status, race, religion, occupation, leisure-time interests, educational level are all factors that will influence the client-counselor relationship. In turn, and possibly of more importance, each of them will affect the type of progress the individual client makes.

* * *

Reaching an agreement on counseling goals is the first step in the development of rapport between the client and the counselor.

Keystones Related to Counseling Skills, Techniques, and Goals

With some clients (e.g., the depressed), frequent, brief sessions may be more practical and productive than full sessions once a week.

* * *

A client may have all the facts, but need counseling to show him where he has distorted some of the data.

* * *

Sometimes a client appears to feel less anxious, in response to a temporary environmental change (e.g., rigid parents go on a vacation and leave student-client home). The counselor might consider this an ideal time to deal with sensitive material that could not be discussed under normal circumstances.

* * *

Having a client list his past accomplishments—ostensibly to obtain background data on him—may help to bolster his self-image at a time when he feels quite inadequate.

* * *

The advantage of having a client give his (subjective) account of the relationships he has had with the significant people in his life is that during such an account his peculiar guilts, defense mechanisms, insecurities, prejudices, and talents come to light.

* * *

In structuring the session, the counselor is demonstrating indirectly to the client the need for discipline and organization in dealing with his complaint.

* * *

When helping the client to recognize the parameters and etiology of a problem, the counselor should first aid him to reject the simplistic view that its source is either *totally* centered in himself or the environment.

* * *

Every environment is limiting to some extent. Yet, progressive fulfillment within its confines is possible if the person realizes his position is not hopeless; if he is willing to invest effort in self-understanding; and if he has the courage to overcome the small frustrations in life, which are the price of enjoying its greater offerings. This message must be understood by every client.

* * *

Resentment is a form of resistance. If the counselor encounters it, she should review the session to see if she has said something to offend the client, or to determine if the pace of the session is too fast.

* * *

When a client sees his problems as indefinable, pervading, or intangible, he may waste his energies in dealing with his general anxieties, fears, self-doubts, and depression. Yet, once he has been helped to relate his difficulties to definite causes, he can begin to take positive steps to alleviate the problems.

* * *

Structuring is a continuing process in counseling. At intervals almost all clients need to be reinformed about the goals, limits, and general methods of counseling.

* * *

By helping the client to effectively deal with a minor problem early in counseling, the counselor sets up the climate that will eventually help him to deal with his more serious difficulties.

* * *

Too much support and reassurance can lead the client to terminate counseling too early.

* * *

Showing interest in what the client says by listening attentively and remembering the small things he says is one way to reinforce communication. Allowing the person to speak without verbally or nonverbally passing judgment on what he says is another.

* * *

Counseling should help rigid clients, who see most of their problems as dilemmas, to become flexible and strong enough to develop new ways of solving their problems.

* * *

One of the objects of counseling is to help the client to master anxiety rather than to avoid situations that cause it.

*   *   *

If a counselor interprets too quickly or exclusively emphasizes a client's liabilities, the client may become defensive and ultimately decide to terminate before making any progress.

*   *   *

At the end of the initial session, the counselor should have (1) given the client an idea of the structural style of counseling that will be used, (2) started to form a basic relationship with the client, and (3) uncovered the primary perceptions the client has of the counselor's role and the expectations the client has in connection with the counseling process.

*   *   *

General inspirational pep talks have no place in counseling. The client must be given concrete support.

*   *   *

Assimilating new information takes time. Therefore, it is not surprising that a client does not immediately understand or accept new concepts proposed by the counselor. He needs several weeks at least to reflect on them before making a real value judgment.

*   *   *

The confusion of decision making is lessened when a person is able to organize his findings into three categories: (1) general goals, (2) potential specific alternative methods, and (3) real limitations.

*   *   *

One of the overall objectives of counseling usually is the replacement of unrealistic goals with rational, attainable ones.

*   *   *

The client must understand that *all* issues can never be resolved in counseling or in life.

*   *   *

Problems become challenges when a person has a positive outlook. Moreover, when problem solving is viewed positively, anxiety does not impede efficiency.

*   *   *

Pain and fear are felt more intensely, and thus have a greater effect on a person, during a period of developmental change. Therefore, the goal of counseling may sometimes be to support the client during these times of transition.

*   *   *

As an educative process, counseling must not only teach the client to recognize his problems, but also to survey the potential solutions available, so that he can ultimately choose a workable one.

* * *

Apathy is a worse problem than anxiety.

* * *

If the client has no objectives when participating in a counseling session, there is no session.

* * *

Counseling may not help a person to control his environment, but it will aid him to better understand and respond to it.

* * *

Counseling may not change *what* a person experiences outside the counseling hour, but it should alter *how* a person experiences life.

* * *

For the client, counseling should be a launching pad to continuing growth. When a client's formal sessions with a counselor are terminated, he should be made to realize that his search for self-fulfillment is a never-ending process.

* * *

Referrals can be as misleading as they are helpful. This is natural since the people who make them are bound by their own opinions, biases, and perceptions.

* * *

The apparently obvious difficulties a person is experiencing may be obscure to him. In reflecting with a client about his characteristic ways of dealing with the world, little should be taken for granted concerning his current level of self-awareness.

* * *

Speed in a counseling session does not parallel progress; usually, the faster the pace, the less achieved.

* * *

Timing is extremely important. *When* the counselor says something is just as crucial as *what* she says.

* * *

No form of counseling is equally effective with all types of people. Likewise, no interviewing or counseling technique is so inviolate that it cannot be modified with a client.

* * *

On certain issues, the counselor may gain insight into the client's true feelings only through careful observation of his nonverbal communications when he is discussing the matter.

* * *

If the counselor can learn what a client daydreams, she may gain a good deal of insight into the client's desires, goals, and values.

* * *

Anxiety prevents a person from organizing his thoughts and priorities. If anxiety can be lowered, it becomes possible to consider previously clouded and feared solutions.

* * *

The counseling process should aid the client to refine his observations of himself and his environment.

* * *

Receptivity to being guided in the pursuit of self-awareness is an intermediate goal of counseling. Development of a desire and an ability in the client to increase his self-awareness on his own is an ultimate goal.

* * *

The more at ease a client becomes with the counselor, the more he will relate to her as he does to other people in his life. So, although the counseling setting is artificial, it still can become a living environment in which the client is able to interact.

* * *

One of the primary and difficult aims of counseling is to transform the client's general feelings into specific questions, problems, and goals.

* * *

Clients can become confused quite easily. Too many issues dealt with in a short span of time may result in one of them being handled improperly.

* * *

When, for some reason, counseling can only consist of several sessions, progress still can be realized. Providing the individual an impetus to change is one accomplishable goal of short-term counseling.

* * *

In counseling, the client's individuality is drawn out so that he can see the traits that set him apart from others.

* * *

Permitting *repeated* negative self-verbalizations by the client serves no positive purpose. Without disagreeing with him, the counselor can (1) ask him to provide specific reasons for such protestations, (2) suggest he explore his positive traits instead, or (3) request him to relate how other people react to him when he speaks in such strong negative terms about himself.

* * *

Compound questions cause confusion. If an issue needs clarification, one—or a series of—short questions should be used, even with the most intellectually advanced clients.

* * *

A question is to a symptom as a group of questions is to a syndrome. Each question should have a specific purpose; each group of questions should form a specific pattern.

* * *

The goal of counseling is often centered on the need for a client to *regain* control over himself and his destiny. In this instance, counseling often need only be short-term since the objective is to aid the client to work through a temporary problem.

* * *

Insight *may* be considered to be an important goal in counseling, but it is not an end in itself. The presence of "enlightened alcoholics" and "aware neurotics" in the community attest to this fact.

* * *

Without a purpose, counseling becomes conversation. And though conversation may be enjoyable for both the counselor and the client, it is a process that will not ultimately prove as fruitful as counseling.

* * *

When a client asks a question or seeks advice, often he already has an answer or solution he thinks is appropriate. Therefore, before making a statement the counselor should redirect the question back to the client to find out his point of view.

b / glossary of psychological and psychiatric terminology

adaptive functioning   term employed in DSM III that is intended to gauge how well an individual is meeting the demands of his/her particular life situation

affect   mood or emotional level

anxiety neurosis   type of neurosis in which anxiety is the central symptom

asthenic reaction   neurotic reaction, formerly termed "neurasthenia," which is characterized by chronic fatigue and listlessness

basic id   form of multimodal therapy devised by Arnold Lazarus that emphasizes seven related but distinct aspects of a person's life: behavior, affect, sensations, imagery, cognition, interpersonal relationships, and drugs (or biological influences)

castration anxiety   anxiety produced by fantasized fear of loss of, or injury to, genitals

compensation   the substitution or exaggeration of something available, for something that is unacceptable or unattainable

countertransference   psychoanalytic term for the development of a transferential reaction toward a patient by a therapist

defense mechanism   unconscious mechanism that a person uses for adaptation

delusion   systematized false belief

differential diagnosis   process of discriminating between similarly appearing symptom patterns

displacement   redirection of emotion from one subject to a more acceptable one

dyad   pair

ego   psychoanalytic term for that portion of the personality that operates according to the dictates of reality

electroconvulsive treatment (ECT) or electroshock treatment (EST)   use of shock by electric current to induce convulsive seizures, as a method of treating certain types of psychoses (i.e., depression)

empathy   the ability to understand and share the feelings of another human being

free-floating anxiety   severe, generalized, persistent anxiety

functional disorder   psychopathological disorder; disorder *without* physical basis

hallucination   sensory experience without physical stimulus or basis

hypomania   mild form of excitement in manic-depressive reaction

id   psychoanalytic term for that part of the personality concerned with immediate gratification of bodily impulses

involutional melancholy   psychotic reaction characterized by depression and agitation

manic-depressive reaction   psychotic reaction characterized by mood swings between elation and depression; often this psychosis takes the form of either one mood or the other

neurasthenia   see "asthenic reaction"

neurologist   medical doctor specializing in the treatment of central nervous system diseases and injuries

passive-aggressive reaction   reaction in which aggression is expended by the person through pouting, stubbornness, and expressions of inefficiency

phobia   persistent, irrational fear

postpartum psychosis   psychotic episode occurring following childbirth

primary prevention   a concept implying the taking of measures to keep people from developing emotional/behavioral disorders

projection   attributing to others one's own (usually) undesirable traits or impulses

projective test   personality test in which the subject is provided with a normally vague stimulus and asked to interpret or structure it; the subject's verbal or written responses are then interpreted by the examiner according to a particular theory of personality

psychiatric social worker   social work specialist concerned primarily with the mentally disturbed

psychiatrist   medical doctor specializing in the diagnosis, prevention, and treatment of mental illness

psychoanalyst   psychiatrist, psychologist, or other senior behavioral scientist with a doctoral degree, who has obtained additional training in a special type of psychotherapy first formulated by Sigmund Freud; to be an analyst, the professional must be analyzed

psychodynamics   theory of human behavior that accepts the presence of unconscious forces and determinism

psychologist (clinical)   academically trained professional normally possessing a doctorate level degree (Psy.D., Ph.D., Ed.D.) and concerned with the diagnosis, prevention, and treatment of mental illness

psychoneurosis (neurosis)   functional disorder in which the person uses defense mechanisms to an exaggerated degree, but does not lose contact with reality or demonstrate gross personality disorganization

psychopathological disorder   syndromes marked by physical symptoms resulting from functionally caused stress

psychopharmacology   study of interaction of drugs with human behavior, particularly in the treatment of emotional stress or disorders

psychosis   severe personality disorder in which there is frequent loss of contact with reality and a gross personality disturbance

rationalization   offering excuses for one's unacceptable behavior or thoughts

reaction formation   demonstration of behavior that is directly opposite to that held unconsciously

regression   a return to a primitive form of behavior as a reaction to stress

reliability   the *consistency* with which a test measures something

repression   unconscious forgetting

re-uptake   the process by which a neuron (nerve cell) reabsorbs the neurotransmitters it has produced

schizophrenia   psychotic thought disorder frequently characterized by withdrawal and emotional flatness or inappropriateness

secondary gain   gain derived from any illness

separation anxiety   fear caused by separation from mother; particularly evident when separation occurs from sixth to tenth month of life

superego   psychoanalytic term for that part of the personality consisting of introjected mores of parents and society

supportive psychotherapy   general type of psychotherapy that uses reassurance, reeducation, and support as a method to bolster the person's current coping and defense mechanisms

symptom   a particular, overt aspect of a disorder

syndrome   group or pattern of symptoms that indicates the presence of a disorder

transference   in psychotherapy, the unconscious identification of the therapist by the patient with someone in the patient's past

unconscious   part of the personality that is not directly accessible to consciousness

validity   extent to which a test measures what it is supposed to measure

chapter references

Introduction

Allen, G., J. Chinsky, S. Larsen, J. Lochman, and H. Selinger. *Community Psychology and the Schools: A Behaviorally Oriented Multilevel Preventive Approach.* Hillsdale, N.J.: Earlbaum, 1976.

Bloom, B. L. *Community Mental Health: A Historical and Critical Analysis.* Morristown, N.J.: General Learning Press, 1973.

Deutsch, A. *The Mentally Ill in America.* New York: Columbia University Press, 1946.

Krasner, L., and L. Ullman, (eds.) *Research in Behavior Modification.* New York: Holt, Rinehart and Winston, 1965.

Meyers, J. "Mental Health Consultation." In *Advances in School Psychology*, edited by T. R. Kratochwill, pp. 133–67. Vol. 1. Hillsdale, N.J.: Earlbaum Associates, 1981.

Meyers, J., R. D. Parsons, and R. Martin. *Mental Health Consultation in the Schools.* San Francisco: Jossey-Bass, 1979.

Moos, R. H. "Conceptualization of Human Environments." *American Psychologist* 28 (1973): 652–65.

———. *The Social Climate Scales: An Overview.* Palo Alto: Consulting Psychologists Press, 1974.

———. *Evaluating Treatment Environments: A Social Ecological Approach.* New York: John Wiley and Sons, 1975.

Parsons, R. D., and J. Meyers. *Consultation Skills: Training, Development, and Assessment.* San Francisco: Jossey-Bass, in press.

Phillips, B. N., R. Martin, and J. Meyers. "Interventions in Relation to Anxiety in School." In *Anxiety: Current Trends in Theory and Research*, edited by C. D. Speilberger. Vol. 2. New York: Academic Press, 1972.

Spivack, G., and M. B. Shure. *Social Adjustment of Young Children.* San Francisco: Jossey-Bass, 1974.

Wolpe, J. *Psychotherapy by Reciprocal Inhibition.* Stanford: Stanford University Press, 1958.

Chapter 1

Egan, G. *You and Me*. Monterey, Calif.: Brooks/Cole, 1977.
Parsons, R. D., and J. Meyers, *Consultation Skills: Training, Development, and Assessment*. San Francisco: Jossey-Bass, in press.

Chapter 2

Detre, T. P., and D. G. Kupfer. "Psychiatric History and Mental Status Examination." In *Comprehensive Textbook of Psychiatry*, edited by A. M. Freedman et al., p. 724. Vol. 1. 2d ed. Baltimore: Williams & Wilkins, 1975.
Lazarus, A. *The Practice of Multimodal Therapy*. New York: McGraw-Hill, 1981.

Chapter 4

American Psychiatric Association. *Diagnostic and Statistical Manual of Mental Disorders (DSM III)*. 3d ed. Washington, D.C.: American Psychiatric Association, 1980.
Szasz, T. *Myth of Mental Illness*. New York: Harper & Row, 1970.

Chapter 5

American Psychiatric Association. *Diagnostic and Statistical Manual of Mental Disorders (DSM III)*. 3d ed. Washington, D.C.: American Psychiatric Association, 1980.

Chapter 6

American Psychiatric Association. *Diagnostic and\Statistical Manual of Mental Disorders (DSM III)*. 3d ed. Washington, D.C.: American Psychiatric Association, 1980.
Beck, A. T. *Cognitive Therapy and the Emotional Disorders*. New York: International Universities Press, 1979.
Burns, D. *Feeling Good*. New York: Signet Books, 1981.

Chapter 7

McBrearty, P. "The Child and Death." *The Forum* (Department of Mental Health Sciences, Hahnemann Medical College and Hospital) 5, no. 1 (1975): 59.
Tyler, L. E. *The Work of the Counselor*, p. 12. New York: Appleton-Century-Crofts, 1961.

Chapter 8

American Psychiatric Association and the National Institute of Mental Health Joint Information Serivce. *The Psychiatric Emergency*. Washington, D.C., 1966.

Caplan, G. *Principles of Preventive Psychiatry*. New York: Basic Books, 1964.

Glass, A. J. "Psychotherapy in the Combat Zone." *American Journal of Psychiatry* 110 (1954): 725–31.

Lindemann, E. "Symptomatology and Management of Acute Grief." *American Journal of Psychiatry* 101 (1944): 141–48.

Menninger, W. C. *Psychiatry in a Troubled World*. New York: Macmillan, 1948.

Querido, A. "The Shaping of Community Mental Health Care." *British Journal of Psychiatry* 114 (1968): 293.

Zusman, J. "Secondary Prevention." In *Comprehensive Textbook of Psychiatry*, edited by A. M. Freedman et al., p. 2335. Vol. 2. 2d ed. Baltimore: Williams & Wilkins, 1975.

Chapter 9

Boenheim, C. "Group Psychotherapy with Adolescents." *International Journal of Group Psychotherapy* 7 (1957): 400.

Steiner, C. *Group Process and Productivity*. New York: Academic Press, 1972.

Yalom, I. D. *The Theory and Practice of Group Psychotherapy*, p. 158. New York: Basic Books, 1975.

Chapter 11

Bennis, W. G. *Organizational Development: Its Nature, Origins, and Prospects*. Reading, Mass.: Addison-Wesley, 1969.

Bergen, J. R. *Behavioral Consultation*. Columbus, Ohio: Merrill, 1977.

Caplan, G. *The Theory and Practice of Mental Health Consultation*. New York: Basic Books, 1970.

Meyers, J., R. Parsons, and R. Martin. *Mental Health Consultation in the Schools*. San Francisco: Jossey-Bass, 1979.

Platt, J., R. Wicks. *The Psychological Consultant*. New York: Grune and Stratton, 1979.

Chapter 12

Dugger, J. *The New Professional: Introduction for the Human Services/Mental Health Worker*. Monterey, Calif.: Brooks/Cole, 1975.

bibliography

Aguilera, Donna C., and Janice M. Messick. *Crisis Intervention: Theory and Methodology*. St. Louis: Mosby, 1974.

Alexander, F. M. *Fundamentals of Psychoanalysis*. New York: W. W. Norton, 1963.

Anderson, Harold H., and Gladys L. Anderson. *An Introduction to Projective Techniques*. Englewood Cliffs, N.J.: Prentice-Hall, 1951.

Appleton, William S., and John M. Davis. *Practical Clinical Psychopharmacology*. New York: Medcom Press, 1973.

Arieti, S., ed. *American Handbook of Psychiatry*. New York: Basic Books, 1975.

Baechler, J. *Suicides*. New York: Basic Books, 1979.

Banaka, William. *Training in Depth Interviewing*. New York: Harper & Row, 1971.

Basmajian, J. V., ed. *Biofeedback—Principles and Practice for Clinicians*. Baltimore: Williams & Wilkins, 1979.

Beck, A. T. *Cognitive Therapy and the Emotional Disorders*. New York: International Universities Press, 1976.

Benjamin, A. *The Helping Interview*. Boston: Houghton Mifflin, 1969.

Benton, Arthur L. "Psychological Tests for Brain Damage." In *Comprehensive Textbook of Psychiatry*, edited by A. M. Freedman et al., pp. 757–68. Vol. 1. 2d ed. Baltimore: Williams & Wilkins, 1975.

Bergantino, L. *Psychotherapy, Insight and Style: the Existential Moment*. Boston: Allyn and Bacon, 1981.

Berkow, Robert, et al. "Tip-offs That You're Dealing with Depression." *Patient Care*, March 1974, pp. 178–85.

Bion, W. R. *Experience with Groups*. New York: Ballantine Books, 1974.

Brill, Naomi I. *Teamwork: Working Together in the Human Services*. Philadelphia: Lippincott, 1976.

———. *Working with People*. Philadelphia: Lippincott, 1973.

Buros, O. *The Mental Measurement Yearbook*. Highland Park, N.J.: Gryphon, 1974.

Caplan, G. *Principles of Preventive Psychiatry*. New York: Basic Books, 1964.

Carr, Arthur C. "Psychological Testing of Intelligence and Personality." In *Comprehensive Textbook of Psychiatry*, edited by A. M. Freedman et al., pp. 736–56. Vol. 1. 2d ed. Baltimore: Williams & Wilkins, 1975.

———. "Some Instruments Commonly Used by Clinical Psychologists." In *Comprehensive Textbook of Psychiatry*, edited by A. M. Freedman et al., pp. 768–71. Vol. 1. 2d ed. Baltimore: Williams & Wilkins, 1975.

Coleman, James C. *Abnormal Psychology and Modern Life.* Glenville, Ill.: Scott-Foresman, 1972.

Cronback, Lee J. *Essentials of Psychological Testing.* New York: Harper & Row, 1960.

DeCato, Clifford M., and Robert J. Wicks. "Psychological Testing Referrals: A Guide for Psychiatrists, Psychiatric Nurses, Physicians in General Practice, and Allied Health Personnel." Unpublished manuscript, 1975.

Dugger, J. *The New Professional: Introduction for the Human Services/Mental Health Worker.* Monterey, Calif.: Brooks/Cole, 1975.

Edwards, D. G. *Existential Psychotherapy.* New York: Gardner Press, 1982.

Ellis, A. *Reason and Emotive Psychotherapy.* New York: Lyle Stuart, 1962.

Ellis, A., and R. A. Harper. *A Guide to Rational Living.* New York: Prentice-Hall, 1961.

Enelow, Allen J., ed. *Depression in Medical Practice.* West Point, Pa: Merck, Sharp & Dohme, 1971.

Fincher, Cameron. *A Preface to Psychology.* New York: Harper & Row, 1964.

Fisher, Walter, Joseph Mehr, and Philip Truckenbrod. *Human Services.* New York: Alfred Publishing Company, 1974.

Freedman, Alfred M., Harold I. Kaplan, and Benjamin J. Sadock, eds. *Comprehensive Textbook of Psychiatry.* 2 vols. 2d ed. Baltimore: Williams & Wilkins, 1975.

Freeman, Frank S. *Theory and Practice of Psychological Testing.* New York: Harper & Row, 1962.

French, J. R., Jr., R. D. Caplan, and R. Van Harrison. *The Mechanism of Job Stress and Strain.* New York: John Wiley and Sons, 1982.

Gartner, Alan. *Paraprofessionals and Their Performance.* New York: Praeger, 1971.

Glasser, W. *Reality Therapy.* New York: Harper & Row, 1965.

Graham, Thomas F. *Mental Status Manual.* East Hanover, N.J.: Sandoz Pharmaceutical, 1973.

Green, Hannah. *I Never Promised You a Rose Garden.* New York: Signet Books, 1964.

Hammer, Emanuel P., ed. *The Clinical Application of Projective Drawings.* Springfield, Ill.: Charles C. Thomas, 1958.

Hayley, J. *Problem Solving Therapy.* New York: Harper & Row, 1976.

Hill, Denis, and Leo Hollister, eds. *The Medical Management of Depression.* New York: Medcom, 1970.

Huber, Jack T. *Report Writing in Psychology and Psychiatry.* New York: Harper & Row, 1961.

Jensen, A. R. *Straight Talk about Mental Tests.* New York: The Free Press, 1981.

Kadushin, Alfred. "Games People Play in Supervision." *Social Work* 13 (1968): 23–32.

———. *The Social Work Interview.* New York: Columbia University Press, 1972.

Kanfer, F., and Arnold Goldstein, eds. *Helping People Change.* New York: Pergamon Press, 1975.

Kaplan, Bert. *The Inner World of Mental Illness.* New York: Harper & Row, 1964.

Kaplan, Harold I., and Benjamin J. Sadock. "Psychiatric Report." In *Comprehensive Textbook of Psychiatry,* edited by A. M. Freedman et al., pp. 733–36. Vol. 2, 2d ed. Baltimore: Williams & Wilkins, 1975.

Keefe, T., and D. E. Maypole. *Relationships in Social Service Practice*. Belmont, Calif.: Brooks/Cole, 1983.

Kerr, M. M., and C. M. Nelson. *Strategies for Managing Behavior Problems in the Classroom*. Columbus, Ohio: Charles Merrill, 1983.

Kolb, Lawrence C. *Modern Clinical Psychiatry*. Philadelphia: Saunders, 1973.

Kosloff, M. A. *Children with Learning and Behavioral Problems*. New York: John Wiley and Sons, 1979.

Levenson, Alan I., and Allan Biegel, eds. *The Community Mental Health Center*. New York: Basic Books, 1972.

Lieb, Julian, Ian I. Lipsitch, and Andrew E. Slaby. *The Crisis Team*. New York: Harper & Row, 1973.

McBrearty, Patricia. "The Child and Death." *The Forum* (Department of the Department of Mental Health Sciences, Hahnemann Medical College and Hospital) 5, no. 1 (1975): 59.

MacKinnon, Roger A., and Robert Michels. *The Psychiatric Interview in Clinical Practice*. Philadelphia: Saunders, 1971.

Magoon, Thomas M., Stuart E. Golann, and Robert W. Freeman. *Mental Health Counselors at Work*. New York: Pergamon Press, 1969.

Martin, William T. *Writing Psychological Reports*. Springfield, Ill.: Charles C Thomas, 1972.

Mathews, Robert A., and Lloyd W. Rowland. *How to Recognize and Handle Abnormal People: A Manual for Police Officers*. New York: National Association for Mental Health, 1954.

Meares, Ainslie. *The Management of the Anxious Patient*. Philadelphia: Saunders, 1963.

Meichenbaum, D. *Cognitive Behavior Modification: An Integrated Approach*. New York: Plenum Press, 1977.

Milton, Ohmer, and Robert G. Wahlers. *Behavior Disorders: Perspectives and Trends*. 3d ed. Philadelphia: Lippincott, 1973.

Nemiah, John C. "Anxiety Neurosis." In *Comprehensive Textbook of Psychiatry*, edited by A. M. Freedman et al., pp. 1198–1208. Vol. 2. 2d ed. Baltimore: Williams & Wilkins, 1975.

Ogdon, D. P. *Psychodiagnostics and Personality Assessment: A Handbook*. 2d ed. Los Angeles, Calif.: Western Psychological Services, 1979.

Panzetta, Anthony F. *Community Mental Health: Myth and Reality*. Philadelphia: Lea & Febiger, 1971.

Patterson, C. H. *Theories of Counseling and Psychotherapy*. New York: Harper & Row, 1973.

Perls, F. S., R. F. Hefferline, and P. Goodman. *Gestalt Therapy*. New York: Harper & Row, 1951.

Rapaport, David, Merton Gill, and Roy Schaefer. *Diagnostic Psychological Testing*, edited by Robert R. Holt. New York: International Universities Press, 1968.

Reiner, Beatrice Simcox, and Irving Kaufman. *Character Disorders in Parents of Delinquents*. New York: Family Service Association of America, 1954.

Rich, John. *Interviewing Children and Adolescents*. London: Macmillan, 1968.

Rimm, D. C., and J. C. Masters. *Behavior Therapy*. New York: Academic Press, 1974.

Rogers, C. R. *Client-Centered Therapy*. Boston: Houghton Mifflin, 1961.

Rowe, Clarence J. *An Outline of Psychiatry*. 6th ed. Dubuque, Iowa: Brown, 1975.

Scaefer, C. E., and H. L. Millman. *Therapies for Children*. San Francisco: Jossey-Bass, 1977.

Scheff, T. J., ed. *Labelling Madness*. Englewood Cliffs, N.J.: Prentice-Hall, 1975.

Seligman, Milton, and Norman F. Baldwin. *Counselor Education and Supervision*. Springfield, Ill.: Charles C Thomas, 1972.

Sneedman, Edwin S., and L. Faberow. *Clues to Suicide*. New York: McGraw-Hill, 1957.

Sobey, Francine. *The Nonprofessional Revolution in Mental Health*. New York: Columbia University Press, 1970.

Stein, M. D., and J. K. Davis. *Therapies for Adolescents*. San Francisco: Jossey-Bass, 1982.

Sullivan, H. S. *Psychiatric Interview*. New York: W. W. Norton, 1952.

Sundberg, Norman D., and Leona E. Tyler. *Clinical Psychology*. New York: Appleton-Century-Crofts, 1962.

Tallent, Norman. *Psychological Report Writing*. Englewood Cliffs, N.J.: Prentice-Hall, 1976.

Tyler, Leona E. *The Work of the Counselor*. New York: Appleton-Century-Crofts, 1961.

Wechsler, David. *The Measurement and Appraisal of Adult Intelligence*. Baltimore: Williams & Wilkins, 1958.

Whittington, H. G. *Clinical Practice in Community Mental Health Centers*. New York: International Universities Press, 1972.

Wicks, Robert J. *Applied Psychology for Law Enforcement and Correction Officers*. New York: McGraw-Hill, 1974.

———. *Correctional Psychology*. San Francisco: Canfield Press, 1974.

Wicks, Robert J., and E. H. Josephs, Jr. *Techniques in Interviewing for Law Enforcement and Corrections Personnel*. Springfield, Ill.: Charles C. Thomas, 1972.

Wolberg, L., ed. *Short Term Psychotherapy*. New York: Grune and Stratton, 1965.

Wolberg, L., ed. *The Technique of Psychotherapy*. 2d ed. New York: Grune and Stratton, 1967.

Wolpe, J. *The Practice of Behavior Therapy*. 3d ed. New York: Pergamon Press, 1982.

World Health Organization. *Prevention of Suicide: Public Health Papers*. Geneva, Switzerland, 1968.

Yalom, Irving D. *The Theory and Practice of Group Psychotherapy*. New York: Basic Books, 1975.

index